INTERNET ADDICTIO

BY

GEETA K. PRAJAPATI (M.A., GSLET, M.ED.)

INDEX

INDEX IN DETAIL

Chapter 01: Introduction

1.1 Introduction

In the present scenario we all know that the Internet Addiction is a burning issue in all over world. Most of people having used internet in Computer, mobile or laptop etc. we all connect to each other via internet, we interact social, educational, entertainment, business and many more thing via internet, this is very easy way for interact to each other, but we have use more internet so we have convert to addiction. So we can say that Internet addiction is a subset of a broader "technology addiction."

Here are a just few advantages that Internet brings to our lives. First of all it provides millions of people with information that is updated by second 24 hours a day, seven day a week. This can play hugely important role in everything from social networking to worldwide stocks and currencies.

With just the click of a mouse you become connected to someone who is another city or even half way across the world. Another advantage is now everyone becomes a genius. That is the Internet has complete change the entertainment. Social networking has also changed that way that friends communicate through the likes of Face book and Twitter. Internet advantages are that internet has completely changed entertainment.

On demand channels now make it possible for us to watch any television programmed that we missed, YouTube lets you search for music video, online news papers. Internet is also using for playing games. People use Internet too much so now they have just addiction about internet.

1.2 What is Internet addiction?

Internet addiction is described as an urge control disorder, which does not engage apply of an exciting drug and is extremely like on the way to pathological gambling. A number of Internet users may increase an emotional affection to on-line associates and actions they produce on their computer screens. Internet users can take pleasure in aspects of the Internet that agree to them to gather meet people, and switch over ideas from side to side the use of chat rooms, social networking websites, or "fundamental communities." Other Internet users expend never-ending hours researching topics of curiosity Online or "blogging".

Blogging is a reduction of the term "Web log", in which a personality will position commentaries and continue usual record of events. Parallel to other addictions, those distresses from Internet addiction use the virtual daydream world to attach with actual people throughout the Internet, as an exchange for real-life human being association, which they are not capable to attain usually. As a model for the description of the IAD he identified the pathological game as Diagnostic and Statistical Manual of Mental Disorders (DSM-IV). The systematic review of the PEU literature has identified the lack of standardization of the concept as an important obstacle to progress in this area of study.

Watching this as a computer game, or watching a video on the Internet which usually find it difficult to interfere with a large number of images or other activities of readers, often divided by online gaming like social activity, Blogging, Email, Pornography or internet shopping(shopping addiction),excessive or inappropriate use of the internet The behavior of anti compulsive behaviors should not be mandatory.

Internet addiction is a detachment of a broader "technology addiction." Widespread mania with skill goes back at smallest amount to radio in the 1930s and television in the 1960s, but in this digital age it is exploded. On ordinary days, largely to allow the intervention measures are provided, social activities such as sports, Internet, video games subcategories of playing or viewing movies or visits to play in trouble on line; Blogs: Mail; There is no or very little kids on the Internet or Internet purchase (procurement). Note that the opponent cannot change the practice and technology of a large group of Internet addiction. Cyber psychology bivauara (2014) in this study, social networks, Internet addiction and began to spread in various countries and is printed on quality of life.

1.3 A Multidimensional Construct

That study recognized seven concepts, or clusters, that create up PIU with a concept mapping move toward. These seven clusters are: psychosocial hazard factors; bodily injury; affecting impairment; social and functional impairment; unsafe Internet use; impetuous Internet use; and Internet use reliance. The last three constructs have not been beforehand recognized.

Uncertain Internet users are behaviors that add to risks of unfavorable penalty. This is not just a tired time on the Internet that puts a young person in danger; there is also an inevitable idea of how much time is spent. The impetuous use build describes an incapability to maintain equilibrium or manage of internet employ in relative to on a daily basis life. Lastly, the reliant use build reflects the added stern symptoms that are characteristically connected with addictions, such as elimination symptoms. Thus, internet addiction might stand for a severe type of PIU.

A variety of facets of Internet employ have to be differentiated for the reason that of their discrepancy predictors, mechanisms and outcome- Online actions which, if complete in person, would usually be measured upsetting, such as obsessive gambling, or shopping, are from time to time called web compulsions.

1.4 DSM Classification for Internet Addiction

Internet addiction disorder is not programmed in the DSM`s present handbook (DSM-5 2013), which is mostly used by psychiatrists. Gambling is a way of conduct disorder (no substance related) is looking at as addiction.

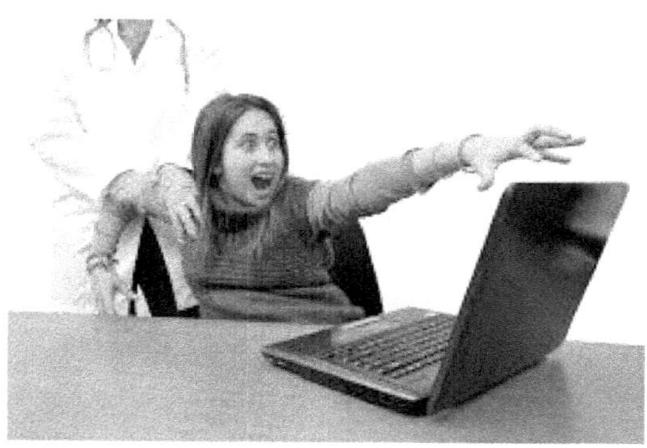

According to Jerald J. Block, M.D. dependency on the Internet is a disorder that should be included in the DSM-5. Although Block observed that it is tough to diagnosis as a disorder because the many symptoms of this addiction are same for other disposable mental health disorder Issues with identifying diagnostic criteria.

The habit to 'cybersex', 'cyber associations, 'net compulsions', 'information and explore and 'computer gaming' are categories explained by Young 1999, that tell to the 'broad' word Internet Addiction. There are a diversity of stimuli online that users could be addicted to quite than the Internet itself, which contain message, gaming, shopping and cyber-relations so some argued that extremely use of internet will increase other addiction too. A study carried out through Young exposed that over half of people measured 'Internet-dependent' were new users of the Internet, and are so additional 'inclined' to use to the Internet regularly It is not easy to notice and make a diagnosis somebody with 'Internet Addiction' as it is a extremely promoted tool'.

1.5 Compulsions Habits for Internet addiction

obsessive online gaming, online gambling, and use of online auction sites are each and every one classed as categories of Internet Addiction, that are supposed to often result in economic and work-related difficulty. Internet users can turn out to be with no trouble addicted to these types of online activity, quite than the Internet itself. The ACE model shows compulsive uses of internet.

Accessibility: Since the expediency of the Internet, users at the present have trouble-free and direct access to gambling, shopping and gaming at any time of day, with no the hassles of daily life (e.g. travelling or queues). Control: Users are in managing of their individual online action. By means of the use of latest technology such as Tablet Computers users can connect with the Internet without knowing other.

Excitement: Internet users excite when they feel of rush or buzz. Gambling, gaming and online bidding every one potentially consequence in succeed. Users will use the net as a technique of gaining this sensation. When internet users get feeling of rush or buzz, they become excite. These online activities are able to generate the emotion of expediency, liberty and thrill, which makes the user desire to perform it once more.

1.6 Internet Addiction and Pornography

Young (1999), The Centre for On-Line Addiction founder claims that Internet addiction is a wide term that covers a broad diversity of behaviors and impulse manage troubles. She claims five specific subtypes counting:

1. Cyber sexual addiction: obsessive make use of adult websites used for cybersex and cyber porn.
2. Cyber-relationship addiction: Over-involvement in online relationships.
3. Net compulsions: compulsive online gambling, shopping or day-trading.
4. Information excess: obsessive web surfing or file searches.
5. Computer addiction: Obsessive computer game playing.

Hyper sexuality has become an enduring focus of empirical consideration in recent years (Kafka, 2010) the study of compulsive Internet pornography use as a sub domain of hyper sexuality has also become a prevalent empirical focus in recent years. In tandem with this increase, the mental health community has witnessed a dramatic rise in problematic Internet pornography use (Manning, 2006; Warden et al. 2004; Owens, Behun, Manning, & Reid, 2012)

According to Joshua B. Grubbs, an expert in Addictive Behavior Patterns, outlines in the journal: Internet Pornography Use: Perceived Addiction, that at current there is no extensively usual means of defining or assessing tricky Internet pornography use and the notion of Internet pornography addiction is still extremely contentious.

1.7 Cyber Relationship Addictions

Cyber-Relationship addiction is related with Internet Addiction Disorder also known as (IAD). It has been supported through different theories and articles over the years such as Ramdhonee's, Psychological impact of internet usage on children and adolescents. A Cyber-Relationship Addiction has been described as, the addiction to community networking inside every forms. Social Networking like Face book, Online_dating_service like Uniform Dating.com are all along among a lot of additional message platforms, creating a position to communicate with new people. Virtual online friends start to gain more communication and importance over time to the person becoming more important than real-life family and friends.

Cyber-Relationships are in essence a virtual relationship or form of communication between two people. Visuals are removed as it is communication through text; all you know of a person is what they are communicating to you and what is displayed on their profile. A person's ambivalence concerning intimacy can be expressed in wording communication since it is a paradoxical mix jointly of allowing people to be truthful and feel close, while as well maintaining their space.

1.8 Issues within Cyber-Relationship Addiction

With the aptitude to make entire fresh personas, people are able to frequently deceive the person they are communicating with. Everybody is looking for the ideal friend but the ideal friend online is not forever the ideal buddy in actual life. Although two people may consign to a Cyber-relationship, offline one of them can not be the individual they are claiming to be present online.

1.9 Fake Personal Profiles People: Chat & Face book (Catfish)

There are people who deliberately create fake personal profiles online with the intention of tricking an innocent person into falling in love with them. These people are known as Catfish. The term Catfish has come from the title of a documentary film released in 2010, in which New York photographer Nev Schulman discovers the woman he'd been continuing a Cyber-Relationship with had not been honest whilst describing herself. From the releases of the film in 2010 Nev Schulman and his team joined up with MTV and created Catfish: the TV Show with the first Season Premiere in 2012.

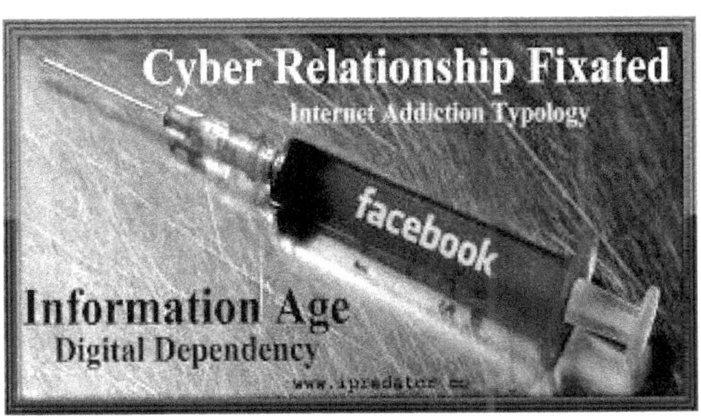

1.10 What are the warning signs of Internet addiction?

Fixation among the Internet (Thoughts regarding earlier on-line action or expectation of the next on-line session Employ of the Internet in growing amounts of time in order to get satisfaction. Frequent, ineffective efforts to control are cut rear or discontinue Internet use. Way of thoughts of annoyance, moodiness, despair, or touchiness when attempting to cut down use of the Internet On-line longer than in the beginning designed. Jeopardized or risked loss of significant relations, occupation instructive or vocation opportunities since of Internet use fabrication to family members, therapists, or others to cover up the degree of participation by the Internet

1.11 How do you use your Internet: Healthy or Unhealthy?

The Internet provides a steady, ever-changing resource of information and entertainment, and be able to be accessed from most smart phones in addition to tablets, laptops, and desktop computers. Although how much is in overindulgence of Internet usage? Every person's Internet use is dissimilar. You may require using the Internet expansively for your occupation, for example, or you may rely a great deal on social networking sites to stay in touch by distant family and friends. Spending a lot of time online just becomes a problem when it absorbs too much of your time, causing you to ignore your relations, your vocation, school, or other vital belongings in your life. If you stay repeating obsessive Internet performance in spite of the negative penalty in your offline life, then it's time to beat a new equilibrium.

1.12 How do citizens turn into enthusiastic to the Internet or Mobile?

Many people turn to the Internet in arrange to handle unlikable feelings like stress, loneliness, depression, and anxiety. When you have a awful day and are looking for a way to run away your troubles or to rapidly reduce tension or self-soothe, the Internet be able to be with no trouble available outlet. Acute uses if online may provisionally create feelings like loneliness, stress; anxiety, depression, and boredom evaporate into thin air. Because much comfort as the Internet can supply, though, it's vital to keep in mind that there are better (and more effective) ways to stay tricky feelings in verify. These can comprise exercising, meditating, and practicing easy relaxation techniques.

For many people, vital feature of overcoming Internet and computer addiction is to discover alternate ways to manage these tricky stances. Yet when your Internet use is rear to strong levels, the sore and unlikable feelings that can have encouraged you to connect in unhealthy Internet use in the past will remain. So, it's worth expenditure some time thoughts about the dissimilar ways you propose to contract with traumatic situations and the everyday irritations that would usually have you logging on.

1.13 Some Risk Factor for Internet Addiction

There are at superior risk of Internet addiction are as under,

You suffer from anxiety. You may use the Internet to sidetrack yourself from your doubts and qualms an anxiety disorder like obsessive-compulsive disorder might also donate to too much email checking and compulsive Internet use.

You are depressed. The Internet be able to be a flee from feelings of misery, but too much time online may create things not as good as. Internet addiction additional contributes to pressure, loneliness and being alone.

You have any other addictions. A most of Internet addicts undergo from further addictions, like drugs, alcohol, gambling, and sex.

You lack social support. Internet addicts frequently use social networking sites, direct messaging, or online gaming as a safe way of establishing new relations and additional self-assuredly connecting to others.

You're an unhappy teenager. You may be wondering where you healthy in and the Internet might feel added at ease than real-life associates.

You are less mobile or socially active than you once were. For example, you might be coping with a new disability those restrictions your capability to drive. Or you might be parenting very little children, which are able to make it tough to depart the house or attach with old associates.

You are stressed. While some people use the Internet to reduce tension, it may have a counterproductive result. The longer you expend online, the higher your tension levels will be.

1.13.1 What are the effects?

Internet Addiction is the result of personal, family, educational, economic and business problems, which are the characteristics of other addictions. Due to excessive use of the Internet, interference in real life relationships is interrupted. Persons anguish from Internet addiction expend extra time in solitary shelter, expend less time with actual people in their lives, and are frequently viewed as socially uncomfortable. Arguments might consequence due to the amount of time used up on-line. Those anguish from Internet addiction might effort to cover up the amount of time spent on-line, which results in disbelieve and the interruption of excellence in once steady relations.

Those at uppermost risk for formation of a concealed life are those who suffer from low-self respect feelings of insufficiency, and fear of condemnation. Such negative self-concepts guide to clinical troubles of misery and anxiety. A lot of persons who effort to give up their Internet use practice removal as well as: anger, depression, relief, mood swings, anxiety, fear, irritability, sadness, loneliness, boredom, restlessness, procrastination, and upset stomach. Internet addiction also results in physical problems or medical problems: Carpal Tunnel Syndrome, dry eyes, backaches, severe headaches, eating irregularities, (such as skipping meals), failure to attend to personal hygiene, and sleep disturbance. Internet addiction also results in physical problems or medical problems:

1.13.2 Causes and Effects:

Dr. Kimberly S. Young says that earlier study associations Internet Addiction Disorder with to be had mental health issues, the majority normally depression. Young states that the disorder has major effects socially, psychologically and occupationally.

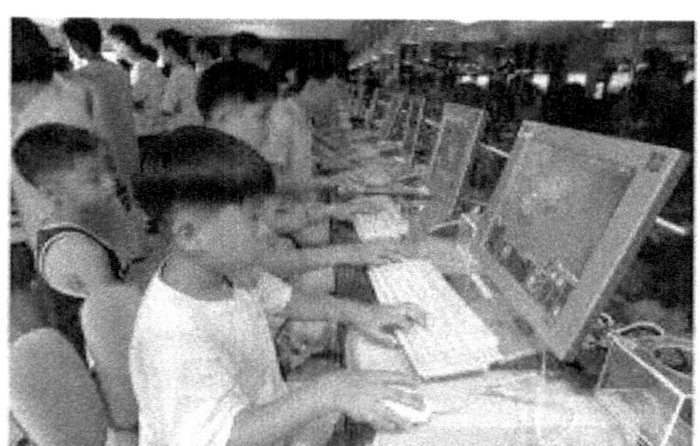

Young states that 52% of the respondents to her own study said that they were following recovery programs for other addictions. These included alcoholism, chemical dependency, compulsive gambling, or chronic overeating. These participants can see the same excessive behaviors, which they need to help in the rest of the internet. Although he believed that the internet addiction is not as seriously as alcoholics, he still felt disappointed that a previous addiction was a new addiction. Young also discusses the findings of Dr. Maressa Hecht-Orzack of McLean Hospital who set of connections a service for computer and Internet addiction in the spring of 1996.

A 2009 study recommended that brain structural changes were present in those classified through the researchers because Internet addicted, comparable to those confidential as chemically addicted. A current study on the effects of online internet gaming reveals how excessive internet addiction could significantly impair a student's brain. For this research, the researchers elected seventeen participants with online gaming addiction and another seventeen naive internet users who hardly ever used the internet.

According to Keath Low, psychotherapist, the orbit frontal cortex, has a big impact on our ability to do things like organizing, prioritizing, focusing on details and remembering and controlling our content. As a result, our online gaming addicts will prioritize their life or to determine the goal and front cover of their classes, focus on planning, priority, focus and remembering the details and controlling our orbit frontal context. There is a big impact on our ability to do things like organizing, prioritizing, focusing on details and remembering and controlling our content.

1.14 Different Internet Addiction Test

The Internet Addiction Test (IAT) of Kimberly Young was the first instrument to assess internet addiction. Initial studies have found that the IAT was a reliable measure that covers the key characteristics of pathological online use. The test measures the extent of a client's involvement with the computer and classifies the addictive behavior in terms of mild, moderate, and severe impairment. The IAT was utilized in outpatient and inpatient settings and adapted accordingly to fit the needs of the clinical setting. The IAT was not validated during its development, but later studies have established its validity in English, and also in Italy and France, making it the first global psychometric measure.

1.14.1 Chen Internet Addiction Scale

The Chen Internet Addiction Scale (CIAS) contains 26 items ranked on a 4-point Likert scale, wherein a higher total score indicates a greater severity of Internet Addiction symptoms. The CIAS was revised to address psychometric properties in adolescents, as well adults. According to the revised edition, 18% of Hong Kong's Chinese teenagers are prevalent in internet addiction.

1.14.2 Compulsive Internet Use Scale (CIUS)

Meerkerk and colleagues was created the Compulsive Internet Use Scale in 2009(CIUS) at the Addiction Research Institute, Rotterdam, Netherlands. It was experienced on two representative samples: 447 serious Internet users, and 16,925 normal Internet users.

The CIUS has 14 items rated on a 5-point scale from 0 = never to 4 = very often. Example item: How often do you find it difficult to stop using the Internet when you are online?

1.14.3 Problematic and Risky Internet Use Scale (PRIUSS)

A newer 18-item measure is the PRIUSS, the Problematic and Risky Internet *Use* Screening Scale, has been developed by Jelenchick and colleagues in 2012 at the University Of Wisconsin School Of Medicine. It is different from this scale that it is based on an experimental model of PIU prepared in the pre-study and during its development the factor has been recognized through development. The instrument is currently being launched in several schools and clinics, as well as being evaluated through further research; it contains 18 items.

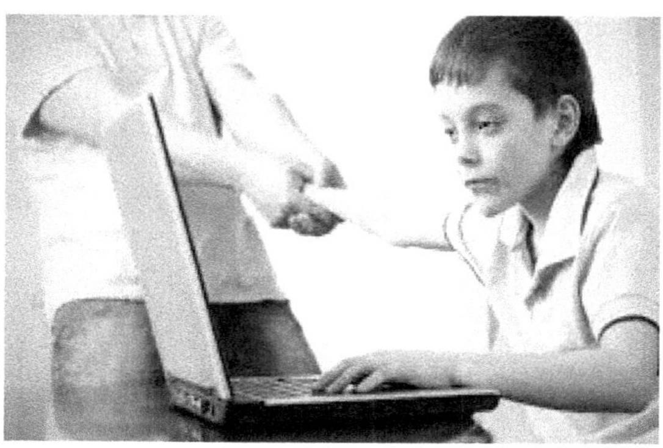

Problematic Internet Use (PIU) is defined as a practice of addiction by strict or poorly controlled fixation, desires or use of computer and work related to Internet connectivity. The current hypothesis for PIU is that individuals prefer online contact for face-to-face connections. Social interaction plays an important role when evaluating time spent on line, as it can develop negative consequences. Looking at PIU, the overuse of the Internet leads to unfortunate health and life consequences. When looking at some of the issues involved when PIU, it is clear that some of these issues are psychosocial variables; they include depression, low self-esteem, loneliness, and shyness. The study found not only the symptoms stated previously but more; such as mood swings, negative outcomes associated with Internet use, compulsive Internet use, and withdrawal symptoms when away from the Internet. The Generalized Problematic Internet Use Scale (GPIUS) has high reliability and validity.

1.15 Mark D. Griffiths Suggested six criteria of Internet addiction are:

1. **Salience:** While the use of the Internet becomes a more important activity in someone's life and his thinking (pre-occupational and cognitive disorders), feelings and behavior (disorder social behavior). For example, even when the person is "off line," they are thinking about the next time they will be on line.

2. **Mood modification:** As a result of the use of the internet, reporting positive people-oriented experiences of people and being seen as a collision strategy for those people (i.e. they "ran away" or "sleep" is a pleasant experience "discussion" or "high.

3. **Tolerance:** The procedure by which users boost the level of Internet use they partake in, to get its mood-modification belongings. There is a propensity to progressively boost the quantity of time spent on line, in order to increase or enlarge those belongings.

4. **Withdrawal symptoms:** Unpleasant feelings and / or physical effects occur when the Internet stops or suddenly decreases. Withdrawal symptoms might include shakiness, moodiness, or irritability.

5. **Conflict:** The various conflicts emerging as a result of the person's excessive Internet use: interpersonal conflict; conflicts with other activities (e.g., job, social life, other

interests); or conflicts within the individual (intrapsychic conflict and/or feelings of loss of control).

6. **Relapse:** Repetition of repetitive repetition, or retrospective behavior patterns, the excessive use of the Internet or the most extreme pattern of intoxication can be quickly restored by the user - even after a period of renunciation or control.

1.16 Different related Internets Disorders are as under:

1.16.1 Online gambling addiction

In Recently a craze for online gambling, it's a very burning issue. According to David Hodgins, a professor of psychology at the University of Calgary, online gambling is considered to be as serious as pathological gambling. It is recognized as an "isolated disorder" which means that persons who have a gambling difficulty favor to divide themselves as of interruptions and distractions. Due to the availability of gambling online, it can increase the problem of bookmakers in social performance, an opportunity to stop gambling without their decision this is the reason that this disorder has more problems on this date and why it is difficult to remove.

The opportunity to gamble online is almost always available in this century opposed to only having the opportunity in a public forum at casinos for example. Online gambling has become quite popular especially with today's adolescents. Today's youth has a greater knowledge of modern software and search engines along with a greater need for extra money. So not only is it easier for them to find opportunities to gamble over any subject, but the incentive to be granted this money is desperately desired.

1.16.2 Stock trading addiction

According to **Brian Bloch** throughout his trading addiction **research** in **July 2013**, online stock trading is one action the image of online gambling that gives a applicant an addictive rush. Online stock trading has an environment that is vulnerable to encouraging addiction. Problem traders have ownership towards when and how they trade stocks and distribute their money. There are no next parties, bosses or schedules so the difficulty trader might automatically feel empowered. Because it is on the Internet, when stock trading, the trader's are able to feel as though they are in their own world and etch out reality.

Bloch explains that it is rather ordinary for difficulty traders to experience "beginners luck" when stock trading, other than because they carry on based off the first rush, they start to misplace wealth After the loss of money, difficulty traders start a cycle of trying to win back their losses which results in an huge financial loss and even insolvency. Your brain produces dopamine when responding to an exciting experience, kind of like your brain is giving your body a reward. By releasing this chemical that gives a pleasurable effect, it is subconsciously teaching the brain that the activity that caused the reaction is positive, and should be repeated. So those who trade stock get a rush when successful and have an "obsessive desire" to repeat the pleasure.

1.16.3 Online gaming addiction (Internet gaming disorder)

In these days Video game addiction is spread in the world. World of War craft has the largest MMORPG (massive multiplayer online role playing games) community on-line and there have been a number of studies about the addictive qualities of the game. Addicts of the game range from children to mature adults. A well-known example is Ryan van Cleave, a university professor whose life declined as he became involved in online gaming. Andrew Doan, MD, PhD, a physician with a research background in neuroscience, battled his own addictions with video games, investing over 20,000 hours of playing games over a period of nine years.

Online gaming addiction might exist measured in terms of B.F. Skinner's theory of operant conditioning, which claims that the incidence of a given behavior is straight linked to satisfying and penalty of that behavior. If behavior is rewarded, it is more likely to be repeated. If it is punished, it becomes suppressed.

Orzack, a clinical psychologist at McLean Hospital in Massachusetts claims that 40 percent of World of War craft (Wow) players are addicted. Orzack explained that the best way to optimize the preferred behaviour in the subject is to give rewards for accurate behaviour, and then regulate the number of times the subject is necessary to display that behaviour earlier than recompense is provided. For example, if a rat must push a bar to take delivery of food, then it will push sooner and additional often if it doesn't know how many times it requirements to force down the bar. The same in World of War craft would be purple (epic) loot drops. Company in World of War craft will often spend weeks hunting for a special item which is based on a chance system, sometimes with only a 0.01% chance of it being dropped by a slain monster.

1.16.4 Communication addiction disorder (Compulsive talking)

Communication addiction disorder (CAD) is a supposed behavioral confusion connected to the requirement of organism in stable communication with additional people, even when there is no realistic requirement for such communication. CAD had been linked to Internet addiction. Users are addictive social fundamentals, such as Facebook and YouTube. Users turn out to be addicted to one-on-one or group message in the form of social support, relations and distraction. However, interference with these activities can lead to conflict and defects. This type of addiction is called the addiction of social network.

Social network addiction is a confidence of people by association, updating and manage of their and their friend's social net page. The correlation between the social network use and a decreasing of offline social relationships is a complex issue, depending not only from the time spent on them but also from the motivation in using them. Sometimes teenagers use social networks to show their ideal image for others. To improve face-to-face relationships, start using social networks in general. However, some of them use these tools as a showcase creating an idealized image to be accepted by groups and to reach a big number of friends. They spend a reduced time for face-to-face relationships, passing instead at least six hours per day on social networks. However, this study reveals that people are using social networks to communicate their real personality and not to promote their idealized identity.

1.16.5 Virtual Reality Addiction

Addiction to virtual reality is an addiction to virtual reality or virtual, immersive environments. At present, interactive virtual media (such as social networks) is referred to as virtual reality, whereas in the future virtual realization is computer-simulated, emersonic environment / world. Experts are comparing the use of Virtual Reality (both in its current and future form) to the use of drugs, bringing with these comparisons the concern that, like drugs, users could possibly get addicted to virtual reality.

1.17 Some general warning signs of Internet Addiction

Signs and symptoms of Internet addiction differ from person to person. For example, there are no set hours per day or number of messages sent that indicate Internet addiction. However at this point are a number of common caution symbols that your Internet use might have turned out to be a trouble?

Losing track of time online: Do you frequently find yourself on the Internet longer than you intended? Do a few minutes turn in to a few hours? Do you get annoyed or crabby if your online time is broken up?

Having trouble completing tasks at work or home: Do you find laundry piling up and little food in the house for dinner because you've been busy online? maybe you discover yourself working behind more frequently since you can't whole your work on time—then staying even longer when everybody also has gone house so you can use the Internet liberally

Isolation from family and friend: Is your social life suffering since of all the time you use up online? Are you neglecting your family and friends? Do you believe like no one in your "actual" life—yet your other half—understands you similar to your online associates?

Feeling responsible or defensive about your Internet use: Are you ill of your other half niggling you to get off the computer or place your Smartphone down and spend time jointly? Do you conceal your Internet use or recline to your superior and family about the amount of time you expend on the computer or mobile devices and what you do while you're online?

Feeling a sense of elation while concerned in Internet actions: Do you apply the Internet as an outlet when worried, depressing, or for sexual satisfaction or excitement? Have you tried to limit your Internet time but failed?

1.18 Physical Symptoms of Internet Addiction

Major 5 symptoms of Internet or computer addiction can also cause physical discomfort such as:

1) Carpal Tunnel Syndrome (pain and numbness in hands and wrists)

2) Dry eyes or strained vision

3) Back aches and neck aches; severe headaches

4) Sleep disturbances

5) Pronounced weight gain or weight loss

1.19 The Treatment of Internet Addiction

1.19.1 Prevention and Treatment

In a lot of cases, even if not all, Internet do to excess corrects itself. Sarah Kershaw wrote for the New York Times in 2005, in reference to Sara Kiesler, professor of computer science and human-computer interaction at Carnegie Mellon University. It was Professor Kiesler who called Internet addiction a craze sickness. In her sight, she supposed, television addiction is not as good as. She added that she was completing a research of serious Internet users, which showed the majority had piercingly reduced their time on the computer in excess of the course of a year, representative that yet difficult use was self-corrective.

Corrective strategies include content-control software, counseling, and cognitive behavioral therapy. One of the major reasons that the Internet is so addicting is the lack of limits and the absence of accountability, Professionals generally agree that, for Internet overuse, controlled use is a more practical goal than total abstinence. Families in the People's Republic of China have turned to unlicensed training camps that offer to "wean" their children, often in their teens, from overuse of the Internet. The training camps have been associated with the death of at least one youth. In November 2009, the government of the People's Republic of China banned physical punishment to "wean" teens from the Internet. Electro-shock therapy had already been banned. In August 2009, Restart, a residential treatment center for "pathological computer use", opened near Seattle, Washington, United States. It offers a 45-day agenda planned to assist people wean themselves from pathological computer use, and may handle up to six patients at a time. In August 2013, researchers at the MIT Media Lab developed a USB-connected keyboard accessory that would "punish" users – with a small electric jolt – who spent too much time on a particular website.

There is a general consensus that total abstinence from the Internet should not be the goal of the interventions and that instead, an abstinence from problematic applications and a controlled and balanced Internet usage should be achieved. The following paragraphs illustrate the various treatment options for IAD that exist today. Unless studies examining the efficacy of the illustrated treatments are not available, findings on the efficacy of the presented treatments are also provided. Unfortunately, most of the treatment studies were of low methodological quality and used an intra-group design.

The general lack of treatment studies notwithstanding, there is treatment guidelines reported by clinicians working in the field of IAD. In her book "Internet Addiction: Symptoms, Evaluation, and Treatment", Young offers some treatment strategies which are already known from the cognitive-behavioral approach: practice opposite time of Internet use (discover patient's patterns of Internet use and disrupt these patterns by suggesting new schedules), (b) use external stoppers (real events or activities prompting the patient to log off), (c) set goals (with regard to the amount of time), (d) abstain from a particular application (that the client is unable to control), (e) use reminder cards (cues that remind the patient of the costs of IAD and benefits of breaking it), (f) develop a personal inventory (shows all the activities that the patient used to engage in or can't find the time due to IAD), (g) enter a support group (compensates for a lack of social support), and (h) engage in family therapy (addresses relational problems in the family) Unfortunately, clinical evidence for the efficacy of these strategies is not mentioned.

1.19.2 Non-psychological Approaches

Some authors have examined medicinal interventions for IAD, it is perhaps the fact that psychopharmacology are used to treat IAD, despite the lack of study of treatment while addressing the efficacy of medicinal healing in the hospital. In particular, selective serotonin-reuptake inhibitors (SSRIs) have been used because of the co-morbid psychiatric symptoms of IAD (e.g. depression and anxiety) for which SSRIs have been found to be effective. Escitalopram (SSRI) was used by Dell'Osso et al. to treat 14 subjects with impulsive-compulsive Internet usage disorder. Internet usage decreased considerably from an average of 36.8 hours/week to a baseline of 16.5 hours/week. In another study Han, Hwang, and Renshaw used bupropion (a non-tricyclic antidepressant) and found a decrease of craving for Internet video game play, total game play time, and cue-induced brain activity in dorsolateral prefrontal cortex after a six week period of bupropion sustained release treatment.

1.19.3 Psychological Approaches

Motivational Interview (MI) is a client-centric yet a client approach that is a guided method to increase internal motivation to find and solve customer's problem. It was developed to help people eliminate the behavior of new behavioral skills, reflective listening, affirmation and summary.

Unfortunately, there is no study of the efficacy of MI in the treatment of IAD, but Mi is effective on average in the field of alcohol, addiction, and diet / exercise problems. Peukert et al suggests that intervention with family members or other relatives, such as "community reinforcement and family training", may be helpful in increasing the motivation of addiction to cut on internet usage, though critics have commented that relatives The studies related to were not present. Reality therapy (RT) should encourage people to change their behavior. It includes sessions to show clients that addiction is an option and is training them in time management; It also offers options for problematic behavior, according to Kim, RT is a major addiction recovery tool that provides many types of experiments in the form of treatment for drug addictions such as drugs, sex, food and internet work. . In the study of the treatment of his RT group consultation program, Kim found that the treatment program effectively reduces the addiction level and increase self-esteem of 25 Internet addicted students in Korea.

Widyanto and Griffith report that most of the treatments employed so far had utilized a cognitive-behavioral approach. The case for using cognitive-behavioral therapy (CBT) is justified due to the good results in the treatment of other behavioral addictions/impulse-control disorders, such as pathological gambling, compulsive shopping, bulimia nervosa, and binge eating-disorders. Wolfing described a predominantly behavioral group treatment including identification of sustaining conditions, establishing of intrinsic motivation to reduce the amount of time being online, learning alternative behaviors, engagement in new social real-life contacts, psycho-education and exposure therapy, but unfortunately clinical evidence for the efficacy of these strategies is not mentioned.

In her research, Young used CBT to treat 114 clients anguish from IAD and establish that respondents were better able to administer their presenting troubles post-treatment, showing enhanced inspiration to discontinue abusing the Internet, enhanced capability to manage their computer use, enhanced capability to function in offline relations, enhanced capability to refrain from sexually explicit online material, enhanced capability to engage in offline activities, and improved ability to achieve sobriety from problematic applications. Cao, Su and Gao, investigated the effect of group CBT on 29 middle school students with IAD and found that IAD scores of the experimental group were lower than of the control group after treatment. The authors also reported improvement in psychological function.

Thirty-eight adolescents with IAD were treated with CBT designed particularly for addicted adolescents by Li and Dai. They found that CBT has good effects on the adolescents with IAD (CIAS scores in the therapy group were significant lower than that in the control group). In the experimental group the scores of depression, anxiety, compulsiveness, self-blame, illusion, and retreat was significantly decreased after treatment. Zhu, Jin, and Zhong compared CBT and electro acupuncture (EA) plus CBT assigning forty-seven patients with IAD to one of the two groups respectively. The authors found that CBT alone or combined with EA can significantly reduce the score of IAD and anxiety on a self-rating scale and improve self-conscious health status in patients with IAD, but the effect obtained by the combined therapy was better.

1.19.4 Multimodal Treatments

A multimodal treatment approach, in some cases, different types of treatments, such as pharmacology, psychotherapy and family counseling, are characterized by many different types of treatments simultaneously or sequentially. Orzack and Orzack mentioned that treatments for IAD need to be multidisciplinary including CBT, psychotropic medication, family therapy, and case managers, because of the complexity of these patients' problems.

In their treatment study, Du, Jiang, and Vance found that multimodal school-based group CBT (including parent training, teacher education, and group CBT) was effective for adolescents with IAD (n = 23), particularly in improving emotional state and regulation ability, behavioral and self-management style. The effect of another multimodal intervention consisting of solution-focused brief therapy (SFBT), family therapy, and CT was investigated among 52 adolescents with IAD in China. After three months of treatment, the scores on an IAD scale (IAD-DQ), the scores on the SCL-90, and the amount of time spent online decreased significantly .Orzack *et al.* used a psycho educational program, which combines psychodynamic and cognitive-behavioral theoretical perspectives, using a combination of Readiness to Change (R.C), CBT and MI interventions to treat a group of 35 men involved in problematic Internet-enabled sexual behavior (IESB). In this group treatment, the quality of life increased and the level of depressive symptoms decreased after 16 (weekly) treatment sessions, but the level of problematic Internet use failed to decrease significantly.

Internet addiction connected symptom scores considerably decreased after a group of 23 middle school pupils with IAD were treated with Behavioral Therapy (BT) or CT, detoxification treatment, psychosocial rehabilitation, personality modeling and parent training. Therefore, the authors concluded that psychotherapy, in particular CT and BT were effective in treating middle school students with IAD. Shek, Tang, and Lo described a multi-level counseling program planned for youthful people with IAD based on the participants of 59 clients. Findings of this study suggest this multi-level counseling program (including counseling, MI, family perspective, case work and group work) is promising to help young people with IAD. Internet addiction sign scores considerably decreased, other than the agenda failed to increase psychological well-being significantly. A six-week group counseling program (including CBT, social competence training, training of self-control strategies and training of communication skills) was shown to be effective on 24 Internet-addicted college students in China The authors reported that the adapted CIAS-R scores of the experimental group were significantly lower than those of the control group post-treatment.

1.19.5 Therapy and Counseling for Internet Addiction

Therapy can give you considerable boost in controlling internet usage. Cognitive-behavioral therapy provides step-by-step methods for preventing binding internet behavior and changing your perceptions regarding internet, smartphone and computer use. Therapy can help you learn the healthy ways of coping with uncomfortable feelings like stress, anxiety or depression.

If your internet usage is directly affecting your partner, with a lot of cybersex or online issues, marriage counseling can help you work through these challenging issues. If you are using the Internet for all your social needs, marriage counseling can help you re-engage with your partner. To help find a therapist for internet addiction, also look at resources as well as a part of the references.

1.19.6 Group Support for Internet Addiction

As internet addiction is relatively new, it can be hard to find a real life support group devoted to issues like Alcoholics Anonymous or Gambler Anonymous. If that is a simultaneous difficulty for you, but, presence groups may help you occupation through your alcohol or gambling troubles as well.

There might as well be groups where you may work on social and coping skills, for example anxiety or depression. There are some Internet Edition support groups on the Internet, however, they should be used with caution. Although you can be directed and helpful in the right direction, you need real life persons to get benefit from relative support.

1.19.7 Helping a Teen an Internet Addiction

It's a fine line as a close relative. If you strictly limit a child or teen's Internet use, they may insurgent and go to overload. But you are supposed to check computer and Smartphone use, oversee online activity, and get your child help out if he or she wants it. If your child or teen is seeing a cryptogram of internet addiction, you can help him: If your child or teen is seeing a cryptogram of internet addiction, you can help him

Encourage other interests and social activities. Take your child out of the computer screen to introduce other hobbies and activities, such as team sports, scouts, and afterschool clubs to children.

Monitor computer usage and set clear limits: control the use of computers or tablets to a general part of the home where you may stay an eye on your child's online action, and limit time online. This will be most effective if you follow to be consistent as parents. If you cannot stay offline, then it is likely that your child will not be either.

Use apps to limit your child's Smartphone use. If your child has his or her individual Smartphone, it's extremely hard to straight observe their time on the Internet.

Further third-party apps are also on hand that get rid of texting and emailing capabilities at the same time as in motion, so you may put off your teen using a Smartphone even as driving. Observe Resources & References part beneath for more information.

Talk to your child about underlying issues. Compulsive computer use can be the sign of deeper problems. Is your child having problems fitting in? Has there been a new most important modify, similar to a shift or separation, which is causing tension?

1.19.8 Do Modify Style of Internet Addiction

To help you see the problem areas, log out how much you use the Internet for non-functioning or unnecessary activities. Are there times of daylight hours so as to you make use of the Internet more? Are there triggers in your day that make you stay online for hours at a time when you only planned to stay for a few minutes? set goals for when you can use the Internet. Replace your Internet usage with healthy activities. If you are bored rigid and feeling alone, resisting the advice to get back online may be extremely hard.

1.20 Review for some Prevalence and supportive internet studies

Over the earlier period decade, the idea of Internet addiction has full-grown in terms of taking as a genuine clinical disorder often requiring action. There is also discussing over whether it should be confidential as an impulse-control disorder or an obsessive-compulsive disorder quite than an addiction. While the survival of Internet addiction is debated, self-proclaimed sufferers are resorting to the courts for redress. In single American case, the plaintiff argued he was unlawfully dismissed as of his service in infringement of the Americans with Disabilities Act because of Internet addiction triggered by means of Vietnam War-related post-traumatic stress disorder (PTSD). the case was dismissed by the United States District Court for the Southern District of New York and affirmed on appeal to the United States Court of Appeals, Second Circuit in 2010 (case summarized in Glaser & Carroll, 2007)

According to research by Kathy Scherer, a psychologist from the The University of Texas at Austin says"13% of college internet users healthy the criteria for Internet addicts" (Scherer 1997). In her study, Scherer enlisted the help of 531 college students. She discovered that "72% of the Internet addicted students were men, (Scherer 1997). The China

Communist Youth League claimed in 2007 that over 17% of Chinese citizens between 13 and 17 were addicted to the Internet. The Internet has wonderful possible to affect the feelings of humans and in turn, modify our self-perception and nervousness levels.

According to Maressa Orzack, director of the Computer Addiction Study at Harvard University's McLean Hospital, between 5% and 10% of Web surfers suffer some form of Web dependency. According to the Center for Internet Addiction revival (whose director is Kimberly S. Young, an investigator who has lobbied for the recognition of network cruelty as a distinct clinical disorder), "Internet addicts suffer from emotional problems such as depression and anxiety-related disorders and often use the fantasy world of the Internet to psychologically escape unpleasant feelings or stressful situations" More than half are also addicted to alcohol, drugs, tobacco, or sex.

Mark Griffiths states that "the way of determining whether nonchemical (i.e., behavioral) addictions are addictive in a no metaphorical sense is to compare them against clinical criteria for other established drug-infested addictions", and although his data is dated, and may no longer represent average Internet use accurately, Griffiths comes to the conclusion that the Internet does meet that criteria for addiction in a small number of users. Scientists have found that compulsive Internet use can produce morphological changes in the structure of the brain. A study which analyzed Chinese college students who had been classified as computer addicts by the study designers and who used a computer around 10 hours a day, 6 days a week, found reductions in the sizes of the dorsolateral prefrontal cortex, rostral anterior cingulated cortex, supplementary motor area and parts of the cerebellum compared to students deemed "not addicted" by the designers. It has been theorized that these changes reflect learning-type cognitive optimizations for using computers more efficiently, but also impaired short-term memory and decision-making abilities—including ones in which may contribute to the desire to stay online instead of be in the real world.

Patricia Wallace PhD, Senior Director, Information Technology and CTY Online, at the Johns Hopkins University Center for Talented Youth argues that based on the case histories that have surfaced, no one denies that excessive involvement with certain psychological spaces on the net can have serious effects on a person's life. She explains that, at a large university in New York, the dropout rate among freshmen newcomers rose dramatically as their investment in computers and Internet access increased, and the administrators learned that 43% of the dropouts were staying up all night on the Internet.

1.21 Mental Health

Mental health includes our emotional, psychological, and social well-being. It affects how we believe, experience, and do something It as well helps determine how we grip tension, narrate to others, and create choices. Mental health is important at every stage of life during childhood and adolescence.

Mental health is a stage of psychological well-being, or an nonattendance of a mental disorder, it is the "psychological state of someone who is functioning at a satisfactory level of emotional and behavioral adjustment", From the viewpoint of positive psychology or holism, mental health might comprise an individual's capability to take pleasure in life, and generate a balance between life behavior and hard work to get psychological resilience. According to World Health Organization (WHO) mental health includes "subjective well-being, perceived self-efficacy, autonomy, competence, intergenerational dependence, and self-actualization of one's intellectual and emotional potential, among others." WHO further states that the well-being of an individual is encompassed in the realization of their abilities, coping with normal stresses of life, productive work and contribution to their community? Though, cultural differences, subjective assessments, and rival expert theories all have an effect on how "mental health" is definite.

A someone stressed with his or her behavioral health might face stress, depression, anxiety, relationship troubles, grief, addiction, ADHD or learning disabilities, mood disorders, or other psychological concerns. Counselors, therapists, life coaches, psychologists, nurse practitioners or physicians may help out deal with behavioral health concerns with treatments like therapy, counseling, or medication. The latest field of global mental health is "the area of study, research and practice that places a main concern on improving mental health and achieving evenhandedness in mental health for every citizen worldwide". Various mental health clinics are now well-known by the phrase behavioral wellness.

1.22 History of Mental Health

In the mid-19th century, William Sweetser was the first to coin the term "mental hygiene" which can be seen as the precursor to contemporary approaches to work on promoting positive mental health. Isaac Ray, one of the thirteen founders of the American Psychiatric Association, further definite mental hygiene since an art to protect the mind aligned with incidents and influences which would reduce or wipe out its energy, quality or progress.

Dorothea Dix (1802–1887) was a vital figure in the progress of "mental hygiene" movement. Dix was a school teacher who endeavored throughout her life to help those suffering from mental illness, and to bring to light the deplorable conditions into which they were put. This was known as the "mental hygiene movement" Before this movement, it was not uncommon that people affected by mental illness in the 19th century would be considerably neglected, frequently left unaccompanied in terrible conditions, hardly even having enough clothing.

Dix's efforts were so great that there was a rise in the number of patients in mental health facilities, which sadly resulted in these patients getting fewer concentrations and be concerned, as these institutions were mainly shorthanded. At the starting of the 20th century, Clifford Beers founded the National Committee for Mental Hygiene and opened the initial outdoor patient mental health clinic in the United States of America. The mental hygiene movement, connected to the social hygiene movement, had at times been connected with advocating eugenics and sterilization of those careful too mentally poor to be assisted into creative vocation and comfortable family life.

Subsequent to year 1945, references to mental hygiene were regularly replaced by the term 'mental health' Evidence from the World Health Organization suggests that almost half of the world's populations are affected by mental sickness with an impact on their self-esteem, relations and capability to role in on a daily basis life. An individual's emotional fitness may also collision physical health and deprived mental health may direct to troubles such as substance abuse.

Maintaining good mental health is crucial to living a long and healthy life. Good mental health may improve one's life, while poor mental health may put off someone from living an elevating life. According to Richards, Campania, & Muse-Burke (2010) that There is growing confirmation that is viewing emotional capabilities are connected with prosaically behaviors like stress management and physical health (2010). It was also completed in their study that people who are short of emotional expression are disposed to anti-social behaviors. These behaviors are a direct indication of their mental health. Self-destructive acts may take place to suppress emotions. Some of these acts include drug and alcohol abuse, physical fights or vandalism.

1.23 Mental Health and well-being

Mental health can be seen as an unstable continuum, where an individual's mental health might have a lot of diverse likely ethics. Mental wellness is in general viewed as a positive characteristic, yet if the individual does not have at all diagnosed mental health situation. This definition of mental health highlights emotional well-being, the capability to live a filled and creative life, and the elasticity to contract with life's expected challenges. Several discussions are formulated in terms of satisfaction or happiness.

A lot of therapeutic systems and self-help books present methods and philosophies espousing strategies and techniques vaunted as efficient for further improving the mental wellness. Positive psychology is more and more well-known in mental health. An example of a wellness model includes one created by Myers, Sweeney and Witmer. It includes five life tasks—strength or spirituality, work and leisure, friendship, love and self-direction—and twelve secondary tasks—sense of worth, sense of control, realistic beliefs, emotional consciousness and coping, problem solving and creativity, sense of humor, nutrition, exercise, self care, stress management, gender identity, and cultural identity—which are recognized since characteristics of strong performance and a main constituent of wellness. The components offer a means of responding to the situation of life in a method that promotes strong performance. The people of the USA, in its greater part are measured to be mostly not educated on the subjects of mental health one more model is psychological well-being.

1.24 Prevention

Mental health can also be defined as an absence of a mental disorder. Focus is increasing on preventing mental disorders. Prevention is beginning to appear in mental health strategies, including the 2004 WHO report "Prevention of Mental Disorders", the 2008 EU "Pact for Mental Health" and the 2011 US National Prevention Strategy. Prevention of a disorder at a young age may significantly decrease the chances that a child will suffer from a disorder later in life.

1.25 Cultural and Religious considerations

Mental health is a socially prepared and socially defined concept; That is, there are many different ways of visualizing their nature and causes in different societies, groups, cultures, organizations and businesses, who decide to become mentally strong and decide which interventions are right. In this way, uneven professionals will have different cultural, class, political and religious backgrounds, which will break the mechanism implemented by treatment.

Research has shown that there is stigma attached to mental illness. In the United Kingdom, the Royal College of Psychiatrists organized the campaign Changing Minds (1998–2003) to help reduce stigma. Understanding mental health professionals, or already, start the importance of qualification in spiritual diversity and spirituality The American Psychological Association explicitly states that religion must be respected. Education in spiritual and religious matters is also necessary by the American Psychiatric Association

Emotional psychological disorders are a major cause of worldwide disability. Investigating the degree and severity of untreated emotional mental disorders throughout the world is a top priority of the World Mental Health (WMH) survey initiative, which was created in 1998 by the World Health Organization (WHO). "Neuropsychiatric disorders are the leading causes of disability worldwide, accounting for 37% of all healthy life years lost through disease. These disorders are most destructive to low and middle-income countries due to their inability to provide their citizens with proper aid. Regardless of current treatment and rehabilitation for emotional mental health disorders, yet economically privileged societies have rival priorities and budgetary constraints".

The World Mental Health survey initiative has suggested a plan for countries to redesign their mental health care systems to best allocate resources. "A first step is documentation of services being used and the extent and nature of unmet needs for treatment. A second step could be to do a cross-national comparison of service use and unmet needs in countries with different mental health care systems. Such comparisons may help to expose most favorable financing, nationwide policies, and delivery systems meant for mental health care."

The coordinated surveys on emotional mental health disorders, their severity, and treatments were implemented in the aforementioned countries. These surveys assessed the frequency, types, and sufficiency of mental health service utilize in 17 countries in which WMH surveys are complete. The WMH also examined unmet needs for treatment in strata defined by the seriousness of mental disorders. Their research showed that "the number of respondents using any 12-month mental health service was generally lower in developing than in developed countries, and the proportion receiving services tended to correspond to countries' percentages of gross domestic product spent on health care". "High levels of unmet need worldwide are not surprising, since WHO Project ATLAS' findings of much lower mental health expenditures than was suggested by the magnitude of burdens from mental illnesses. Generally, unmet needs in low-income and middle-income countries might be attributable to these nations spending reduced amounts (usually <1%) of already diminished health budgets on mental health care, and they rely heavily on out-of-pocket spending by citizens who are ill equipped for it".

1.26 Organizations

Firstly, Women's College Hospital is especially dedicated to the health of women in Canada. The hospital is located in the heart of downtown, Toronto, where many places are available for certain medical conditions. WCH is a great organization that helps women educate on mental illness due to their expertise with women and mental health. Women's colleges, hospitals help the persons who have mental depression, such as depression, anxiety, menstruation, pregnancy, childbirth, and menopause symptoms. They also focus on psychological issues, abuse, neglect, and mental health related problems from various drugs.

The second organization is the Centre for Addiction and Mental Health. CAMH is one of Canada's largest and most well-known health and addiction facilities. They practice in doing research in areas of addiction and mental health in both men and women. In order to help both men and women, CAMH provides "clinical care, research, education, policy development and health promotion to help transform the lives of people affected by mental health and addiction issues."(CAMH: Who We Are, 2012). As a public hospital, CAMH is known throughout the world as a "Pan American Health Organization and World Health Organization Collaborating Centre"(CAMH: Who We Are, 2012). CAMH is different from Women's College Hospital due to its widely known rehab centre for women who have minor addiction issues, to severe ones. This organization provides care for mental health issues by assessments, interventions, residential programs, treatments, and doctor and family support.

1.26.1 Organization of U.S.

According to the World Health Organization in 2004, depression is the leading cause of disability in the United States of America for individuals ages 15 to 44. Absence from work in the U.S. due to depression is estimated to be in excess of $31 billion per year. Depression frequently co-occurs with a variety of medical illnesses such as disease, cancer, and chronic pain and is associated with poorer health status and prognosis. Each year, roughly 30,000 Americans take their lives, while hundreds of thousands make suicide attempts (Centers for Disease Control and Prevention). In 2004, suicide was the 11th leading cause of death in the United States of America (Centers for Disease Control and Prevention), third among individuals ages 15–24. Despite the increasingly availability of effectual depression treatment, the level of unmet need for treatment remains high. By way of comparison, a study conducted in Australia during 2006 to 2007 reported that one-third (34.9%) of patients diagnosed with a mental health disorder had had presented to medical health services for treatment.

There are many factors that influence mental health including:

- Mental illness, disability, and suicide are ultimately the result of a combination of biology, environment, and access to and utilization of mental health treatment.

- Public health policies may influence admittance and utilization, which subsequently may improve mental health and help to progress the negative consequences of depression and its associated disability.

Emotional mental illnesses should be a particular concern in the United States of America since the U.S.A has the maximum yearly incidence rates (26 percent) for mental illnesses amongst a comparison of 14 increasing and developed countries. While just about 80 percent of all citizens in the United States with a mental disorder ultimately be given some form of treatment, on the normal persons do not access be concerned until virtually a decade next the progress of their illness, and less than one-third of citizens who seek out help be given simply enough be concerned.

1.27 Policies for Mental Health by U.S.

The mental health policies in the United States have qualified four most important reforms: the American asylum association led by Dorothea Dix in 1843; the mental hygiene movement stimulated through Clifford Beers in 1908; the deinstitutionalization in progress by Action for Mental Health in 1961; and the group of people hold up movement called for by The CMCH Act Amendments of 1975.

In 1843, Dorothea Dix submitted a Memorial to the Legislature of Massachusetts, describing the abusive treatment and horrible conditions received by the mentally ill patients in jails, cages, and almshouses. She used to say that they came to remembrance before drawing attention to the people in cages, collages, sellers, shops, pens, and the present mad people in the Commonwealth. Associated, nude, beaten with rods, and lashed in obedience Many asylums were built in that period, with high fences or walls separating the patients from other community members and strict rules regarding the entrance and exit. In those asylums, traditional treatments were well implemented: drugs were not used as a cure for a disease, but a way to reset equilibrium in a person's body, along with other essential elements such as healthy diets, fresh air, middle class culture, and the visits by their neighboring residents. In 1866, a recommendation came to the New York State Legislature to establish a separate asylum for chronic mentally ill patients. Some hospitals placed the chronic patients into separate wings or wards, or different buildings.

In A Mind That Found Itself **(1908) Clifford Whittingham Beers** described the humiliating treatment he received and the deplorable conditions in the mental hospital. One year later, the National Committee for Mental Hygiene (NCMH) was founded by a small group of reform-minded scholars and scientists – including Beer himself – which marked the beginning of the "mental hygiene" movement. The movement emphasized the importance of childhood prevention. World War I catalyzed this idea with an additional emphasis on the impact of maladjustment, which convinced the hygienists that prevention was the only practical approach to handle mental health issues. However, prevention was not successful, especially for chronic illness; the condemnable conditions in the hospitals were even more prevalent, especially under the pressure of the increasing number of chronically ill and the influence of the Depression.

In 1961, the Joint Commission on Mental Health published a report called Action for Mental Health, whose goal was for community clinic care to take on the burden of prevention and early intervention of the mental illness, therefore to leave space in the hospitals for severe and chronic patients. The court started to rule in favor of the patients' will on whether they should be forced to treatment. By 1977, 650 groups of people mental health centers were built to cover 43 percent of the population and serve up 1.9 million persons a year, and the lengths of treatment decreased from 6 months to only 23 days. However, issues still existed. Due to inflation, especially in the 1970s, the community nursing homes received less money to support the care and treatment provided. Fewer than half of the planned centers were created, and new methods did not fully replace the old approaches to carry out its full capacity of treating power. Besides, the community helping system was not fully established to support the patients' housing, vocational opportunities, income supports, and other benefits. Many patients returned to welfare and criminal justice institutions, and more became homeless. The movement of deinstitutionalization was facing great challenges.

subsequent to realizing that just changing the site of mental health care from the state hospitals to nursing houses was not enough to put into practice the idea of deinstitutionalization, the National Institute of Mental Health in 1975 shaped the Community Support Program (CSP) to supply finances for communities to set up a inclusive mental health service and ropes to help the mentally ill patients put together productively in the society. In addition, the Congress enacted the Mental Health Systems Act to prioritize the service to the mentally ill and emphasize the expansion of services beyond just clinical care alone. Later in the 1980s, under the influence from the Congress and the Supreme Court, many programs started to help the patients regain their benefits. A new Medicaid service was also established to serve people who were suffering from a "chronic mental illness." People who were temporally hospitalized were also provided aid and care and a pre-release program was created to enable people to apply for reinstatement prior to discharge. Not until 1990, around 35 years after the start of the deinstitutionalization, did the first state hospital begin to close. The number of hospitals dropped from around 300 by over 40 in the 1990s, and finally a Report on Mental Health showed the efficacy of mental health treatment, giving a range of treatments available for patients to choose.

The 2011 National Prevention Strategy incorporated mental and emotional well-being, with recommendations as well as better parenting and near the beginning interference programs, which boost the probability of avoidance programs organism incorporated in future US mental health policies. The NIMH is researching only suicide and HIV/AIDS prevention, but the National Prevention Strategy could lead to it focusing more broadly on longitudinal prevention studies.

1.28 Emotional Improvement

Being mentally and emotionally healthy does not prevent the experiences of existence which we cannot manage. As humans we are going to face emotions and events that are a part of life. According to Smith and Segal that public who are emotionally and mentally healthy have the tools for coping with tricky situations and maintaining a constructive viewpoint in which they also stay put listening carefully, flexible, and inspired in bad times as well as good(2011). In addition unemployment has been shown to have a negative impact on an individual's emotional well-being, self-esteem and more broadly their mental health. Increasing unemployment has been show to have a significant impact on mental health, predominantly depressive disorders. This is a vital deliberation when reviewing the triggers for mental health disorders in several population surveys. In order to improve your emotional mental health, the root of the issue has to be resolved. Prevention emphasizes the escaping of danger factors; encouragement aims to improve an individual's capability to realize a positive sense of self-esteem, mastery, well-being, and social inclusion (Power, 2010).

It is very important to improve your emotional mental health by surrounding yourself with positive relationships. We as humans, feed off companionships and interaction with other people. Another way to get better your emotional mental health is participating in actions that may permit you to calm down and take time for yourself. Yoga is a great example of an activity that calms your entire body and nerves. According to a study on well-being by Richards, Campania and Muse-Burke that mindfulness is considered to be a purposeful state, it may be that those who practice it believe in its importance and value being mindful, so that valuing of self-care activities may influence the intentional component of mindfulness (2010).

1.29 Mental Health Care Navigation

Mental health care is direction-finding helps to direct patients and families through the fragmented, often baffling mental health industries. Care navigators work closely with patients and families through discussion and collaboration to provide information on best therapies as well as referrals to practitioners and facilities specializing in particular forms of emotional improvement.

The difference between therapy and care navigation is that the car navigation process provides information and directs patients to therapy rather than providing therapy. Still, care navigators may offer diagnosis and treatment planning. Although many care navigators are also trained therapists and doctors. Care navigation is the link between the patient and the below therapies. A clear recognition that mental health requires medical intervention was demonstrated in a study by Kessler et al. of the prevalence and treatment of mental disorders from 1990 to 2003 in the U. S. A. Despite the prevalence of mental health disorders remaining unchanged during this period, the number of patients seeking treatment for mental disorders increased threefold.

1.30 Therapy for Good Mental Health:

1.30.1 Activity therapies

Activity therapies, also called recreation therapy and occupational therapy, promote healing through active engagement. Making crafts can be a part of occupational therapy. Walks may be a fraction of hobby therapy

1.30.2 Expressive therapies

Expressive therapies are a form of psychotherapy that involves the arts or art-making. These therapies include music therapy, art therapy, dance therapy, drama therapy, and poetry therapy.

1.30.3 Alternative therapies

Alternative therapy is a branch of alternative medicine, which includes a large number of therapies imported from other cultures. It also includes a number of new medicines that have not yet passed through the process of scientific review.

1.30.4 Meditation

Increased awareness of mental processes can influence emotional behavior and mental health. A 2011 study incorporating three types of meditative practice (concentration meditation, mindfulness meditation and compassion toward others) revealed that meditation provides an enhanced ability to recognize emotions in others and their own emotional patterns, so they could better resolve difficult problems in their relationships

1.30.5 Biofeedback

Biofeedback is a process of gaining control of physical processes and brainwaves. It can be used to decrease anxiety, increase well-being, increase relaxation, and other methods of mind-over-body control.

1.30.6 Group therapy

Group therapy involves any type of therapy that takes place in a setting involving multiple people. It can include psychodynamic groups, activity groups for therapy, support (including the Twelve-step program), problem-solving and psycho education groups.

1.30.7 Pastoral counseling

Pastoral counseling is the merging of psychological and religious therapies and carried out by religious leaders or others trained in linking the two.

1.30.8 Psychotherapy

Psychotherapy is the universal term intended for scientific based treatment of mental health issues based on contemporary medicine. It includes a number of schools, such as therapy, psychoanalysis, cognitive behavioral therapy and dialectical behavioral therapy.

1.31 Type for Mental Illness:

There are many different conditions that are recognized as mental illnesses. The more common types include:

1.31.1 Anxiety disorders

People with panic disorder respond to specific things or situations with fear and dread, as well as concerns of heart rate and sweating, and signs of anxiety are not suitable for the reaction of the person, if someone does not control the reaction If anxiety interferes with normal functioning, anxiety disorder is diagnosed. Panic disorder includes general anxiety disorders, anxiety disorders, social anxiety disorders, and specific fears.

1.31.2 Mood disorders

These disorders are also called emotional disorders, which include extreme depression or extreme happiness, extreme pleasure and extreme distress. The most common mood disorders are depression, bipolar disorder, and cyclothymiacs disorders.

1.31.3 Psychotic disorders

Psychological disorders include distorted awareness and thinking. The two most common symptoms of psychological disorders are hallucinations - the experience of images or sounds is not realistic, like listening to the voice - and confusion, which is a bogus permanent belief that accepts a sick person due to reality.

1.31.4 Eating disorders

Anorexia nervosa, bulimia nervosa and binge diet disorder are the most common food disorders in excessive emotions, behaviors, and weight and dietary behaviors in food disorders.

1.31.5 Impulse control and addiction disorders

People with desire control disorders are not able to meet the harmful actions themselves or others, or cannot cope with impulses, Pyromania (starting fire), kleptomania (theft), and compulsive gambling impulse control Examples of disorders are: Alcohol and drugs are the common things of addiction Often, people with these disorders turn out to be so concerned with the matter of their addiction that they start on to pay no attention to responsibilities and relations.

1.31.6 Personality disorders

People with personality disorders have extreme and inflexible personality traits that are distressing to the person and/or cause problems in work, school, or social relationships. In addition, the individual's patterns of thoughts and behavior considerably be different as of the expectations of society and are so rigid that they interfere with the person's normal functioning. Examples include antisocial personality disorder, obsessive-compulsive personality disorder, and paranoid personality disorder.

1.31.7 Obsessive-compulsive disorder (OCD)

People with OCD suffer from constant thoughts or fear, which inspires them to do some rites or routines. Sad thought is called, and religious rituals are called compulsions. For example, there is a person who works hard with the fear of microbes, who constantly wash their hands

1.31.8 Post-traumatic stress disorder (PTSD)

A sufferer is a condition that can develop painful and / or horrible events, such as sexual or physical assault, unexpected death of a loved one or a natural disaster. People with PTSD often have permanent thoughts and memories of the event, and are emotionally numbers.

1.32 Importance of Study

This section brings out the various organizations in which the study was undertaken and under which guidance the study was authorized. **Hemchandracharya University, Patan** authenticated the research work and under the guidance of **Dr. C.R.Suchak**. The Research practice and Data collection for Arts, Commerce and Science College Students was undertaken with the help of different college principal and teaching-non teaching staff also. The **Research Sample** of general category from the **Ahemdabad, Gandhinagar, Vishnagar** etc. region and also population of various organizations working in this region have been considered for the study. The group was **randomly selected** by administering the testing inventories. **The library** of **Gujarat University**, The library of **Patan University**, the Library of **Govt. Arts College Gandhinagar** have largely benefited in collection of the historical evidences of Psychology. Its associates have largely contributed in the collection of the data for the research work.

Now after having known the organizations in which the study was conducted, it is essential to understand as to how the study was conducted an overview of the same is brought under: This study has been intended to bring out the differences of Arts, Commerce and Science college students on Internet Addiction and Mental Health. This study is very useful from different field like as: Applied psychology, Social psychology and also community psychology. Last but not least this study high lights in burning issue for our society.

1.33 Organization of Study Materials

So the entire study is divided into **five chapters** and brief description of each chapter is brought down here under:

Chapter 1: Introduction

The first chapter is of the introductory nature dealing with the need of this type of research work and its relevance in the present day context tracing to the historical background of What is Internet Addiction, Type Of Internet Addiction, causes and effects of Internet Addiction, Internet Addiction and related Health problem, what is Mental Health, Type of Mental Illness, W.H.O. definition for Mental Health etc

Chapter 2: Review of Literature

In this chapter various literatures on Internet addiction and Mental Health of college students and also other people was shown. First of all we seen the Review of Literature for Internet Addiction than we seen the Review of Literature for Mental health.

Chapter 3: Research design of the study, Procedures and Method of analysis

The third chapter deals with the research design. It also states how the sample was selected from the population, which sampling method was used and its detailed narration has been discussed. Collection of data, research tools, measurement of independent variables discussed in detail.

Chapter 4: Analysis of the Result, Interpretation and Discussions

This chapter deals with the analysis of the chapter in terms of statistics and the interpretation from the inferences obtained through the statistics. Further, case histories, suggestions for improvement and recommendations are discussed in detail.

Chapter 5: Research Report

This chapter deals with the summary of the research, conclusions based on statistical technique, conclusions regarding all the variables, Recommendations, suggestions for further research are discussed.

Chapter 02: Review of Relevant Literature

2.1. Introduction

The researcher need to acquire up to date information of what has been thought and said in a particular area, so that they can drive benefit from the work of their predecessors. According to Scot & Wertheimer (1992) Review of related literature may help to make progress towards the solution of new problems emphasizing to the importance of survey of related literature. This section chiefly brings out the literature materials which were used as guidelines for the study. Further, this section brings out the topics such as Internet Addiction and Mental Health among the Students of Arts, Commerce and science Faculty Students studies. Now, let us examine each topic under their heads explicitly.

2.2 A Review of Relevant literature for Internet addiction

1) Internet Use among College Students: An Exploratory Study

Keith.J.A. (2010)

In this studies representative sample of 1,300 college students of 8th standard was selected to find out the effect of internet to their social or educational lives. The students who use the Internet for 100 minutes per day, a small group of students employ the Internet to a degree that interferes with other aspects of their lives. Most of them are men. And they are found with the hard science academic majors. Various ideas for dealing with this problem are suggested.

2) Some Observations on Internet Addiction Disorder Research

Prasnna, C.H. & et.al.(2013)

In this research the study indicated that Internet addiction is a contemporary difficulty brings about through trouble-free access to computers and online information. Internet addicted persons can expand many types of disorders. In severe cases, Internet addicted can be harmful to themselves, their families, and their place of employment. Business executives have need of to include a superior considerate of Internet addiction since employees with Internet addiction can be really counter- productive as well as cause other legal problems. This study examines research trends in the area of Internet addiction and provides administration implications in favor of policy expansion and planning. Specially, this study identifies the most important researchers, institutions, specialization, and information distribution outlets for Internet addiction research. This study should be of attention to educators at educational institutions, students interested in institutions offering Internet addiction courses and programs. The different fields of psychology will help to reveal the result of this research. This study results will be valuable for the employees of corporate sector, the department of human resource, computing consultants, and risk assessors of insurance companies will find the results of this study to be valuable.

3) The Investigation between Arts and science Students on Internet Addiction

Savaliya V.M.(2013)

Purpose: To explore significant difference between the students of Arts and science on Internet Addiction

Method: In this research internet addiction questioner were administrated individually used to as well as on male and female students of arts and science faculty in Saurashtra university campus. In a representative sample of 120 students was selected in this research. The tool for internet addiction questioner was developed by Kimbel Young Was used in this research.

Conclusion: Here, the results show that the students of Arts and Science are not same internet addicted. But we can say that Arts students are more Internet Addicted than science students.

4) The association between internet addiction and self-injurious behaviour among adolescents

Lam.L.T.(2009)

Objective: To study the association between internet addiction and self-injurious behaviour (SIB) in adolescence.

Methods: Total sample consisted of 1618 high school students was selected from Guangzhou city. Here SIB was intentional using self-reported questionnaire and internet addiction was examined using the Internet Addiction Test (IAT).

Conclusions: The finding of study revealed that SIB was common in adolescence population in China. Internet Addiction was harsh to mental health and increases the risk of self-injury among adolescents.

5) Internet addiction among private sector employees

Patel A.C. (2015)

Purpose: To examine mean difference between male and female of private sector employees on Internet Addiction.

Method: In this research internet addiction questioner were administrated individually used to as well as on male and female employees of private sector, while after the data collection was completed then **t** test was used to find out mean difference between male and female employees. The research tool of I.A.Q. was developed by Kimbal Young`s, Gujarati version by Mittal Vekariya was used in this research. The total sample consisted of 100 employees, whom 50 are male employees and other 50 are female employees from Ahmadabad city.

Conclusion: The finding of the study revealed that there was no significance mean difference between male and employees of private sector on Internet Addiction. Here male employees are more internet addict than female employees in private sector.

6) A New Clinical Phenomenon and Its Consequences for Internet Addiction

Kimberly S. Y. (2009)

Latest research identifies online users who became hooked on chat rooms, interactive games, and even play only to see their lives become gradually more uncontrollable as the Internet. Former research explores the addictive qualities supporting drug and alcohol misuse, pathological gambling, and even video game addiction; however, given the next of kin freshness of Internet addiction, little is understood about the habit-forming nature of the Internet and it's possible for mouse. In this days our lives at home, school, and works is very affected by internet. This article try to find out how the Internet can create marital-, academic-, and job-related problems.

7) A comparative study of 12th science stream boys and girls on internet addiction

Parmar H.K. (2014)

Purpose: comparative study of 12th science stream boys and girls to find out mean difference on internet addiction.

Method: In this research internet addiction questioner were administrated individually used to as well as on 12th standard boys and girls, while after the data collection was completed then **t** test was used to find out mean difference between boys and girls. In a representative sample of 140 students were selected in this research. The research tool of I.A.Q. was developed by Kimbal Young`s, Gujarati version by Mittal Vekariya was used in this research.

Conclusion: There is a significance mean difference between boys and girls of 12th standard science stream.

8) Does Internet and Computer "Addiction" Exist? Some Case Study Evidence

Griffiths, M.D. (2005)

We can assume that social pathologies are start to surface in cyberspace. To date, there is very little empirical evidence that computing activities are addictive. Some evidence shows that the characteristic of addict is an adolescent, usually male, with little or no social life, and little or no self-confidence. This article was study about five case studies of acute computer usage. Out of the five cases, only two of them explain "addicted' subjects. Addiction components criteria were used in the assessment. The too much usage in the greater part of cases was simply indicative and was highlighted how the subjects used the Internet/computer to counteract other deficiencies.

9) Addiction and physical and psychosocial behavior problems among rural secondary school students

Kamer Gür & et.al (2014)

The main objective was to combat physical and psychological behavioral problems through this study of secondary school students' level and internet addiction internship in this study. In rural area this study was conducted in three state secondary schools in western part of Turkey. Total sample consisted of 549 students who agreed to participate, with the permission of their families, and who had an Internet connection at house. The t-tests and variance analyses were using to calculate the data. In this study most of students get medium level score of Internet addiction (mean addiction score 44.51 ± 17.90). There were remarkable differences between the Internet addiction scores and the presence of physical behavior problems of students(going to bed late, skipping meals, eating meals in front of the computer) and psychosocial behavior troubles (distress from situation for example restlessness, anger, heart palpitations, or tremors when they could not attach through Internet, decreased relationships with family and associates, feelings of anger, in conflict with parents, and finding life boring and blank lacking of an Internet connection.

10) A study of Internet addiction and Mental Hygiene among boys and girls of government engineering college students

Shah H.A. (2014)

Purpose: To examine mean difference between boys and girls of government engineering college on Internet Addiction and mental hygiene.

Method: In this research two tests were administrated individually used to as well as on boys and girls of government engineering college Rajkot, while after the data collection was completed then **t** test was used to find out mean difference between boys and girls on internet addiction and mental hygiene. The research tool of I.A.Q. was developed by Kimbal Young`s, Gujarati version by mittal vekariya was used in this research and Mental hygiene questionerwas developed by Dr.D.J.Bhatt and Gita R.Gida. The total sample consisted of 160 employees, whom 80 are boys and other 80 are girls from Rajkot city.

Conclusion: The finding of the study revealed that there was significance mean difference between boys and girls of government engineering college students on internet addiction and also mental health.

11) Internet Use, Abuse, and Dependence among Students at a Southeastern Regional University

Beverly L.F. (2007)

Objective: To assess Internet use, abuse, and dependence.

Participants: The total sample consist 411 undergraduate students.

Results: in this research 90% of participants reported daily Internet use. Just about 50% of the sample met criteria for Internet abuse, and 25%met criteria for Internet dependence. Men and women did not differ on the mean amount of time accessing the Internet each day; however, the reasons for accessing the Internet differed between the 2 groups. The result saw that depression was correlated with more frequent use of the Internet to meet people, socially experiment, and participate in chat rooms, and with less frequent face-to-face socialization. In addition, individuals meeting criteria for Internet abuse and dependence endorsed more depressive symptoms, more time online, and less face-to-face socialization than did those not meeting the criteria.

Conclusions: Mental health and student-care professionals should be warning of problems related to overuse of the Internet, especially computers become an integral part of college life.

2.3 A Review of Relevant literature for Mental Health

1) The Association between Mental Health and Acute Infectious Illness among a National Sample of 18- to 24-Year-Old College Students

Troy B. A. (2008)

Objective: Underprivileged mental health is related with physical illness, but this connection is badly characterized with college students.

Participants: The authors diagnosed poor mental health (depression, anxiety, and negative effects) and examined the relationship between poor mental health and acute transmissible illness such as bronchitis, ear infections, sinusitis, straps throat etc. among 47,202 US college students.

Methods: A Frequency and cross-tabulation analysis was used to characterize mental health in this study. They used dual logistic regression to determine the association between poor mental health and acute infectious illness, controlling for research-derived covariates.

Results: The number of acute infectious diseases ranges from 8% to 29%. The spread of anxiety and depression was 12% to 20%, respectively. Depression, anxiety and fatigue were associated with severe infections in all the dependent steps, including halts from 0.56 to 0.91.

Conclusions: Poor mental health is related with acute communicable illness among college students.

2) A comparative study of Mental Health among Government and private school teachers

Vyas K.R. (2014)

Purpose: To examine Mental Health among government and private school teachers

Method: Total sample consisted of 80 teachers was selected from Ahmedabad city that 40 were government school teachers and another 40 were private school teachers. The research tool for Mental Health was developed by Dr.D.J.Bhatt and Gita R.Gida was used in this research .Here,t-test was applied to check the significance difference between government and private school teachers.

Conclusion: The finding of the study revealed that there was significance mean difference between government and private school teachers and also found that the mean difference of government school teachers was very high to compare private school teachers.

3) Stigma and Help Seeking for Mental Health among College Students

MarilynF.D.et.al. (2009)

Mental illness stigma has been identified by national policy makers as an important barrier to help seeking for mental health. Total sample consist of 5,555 students from a diverse set of 13 universities, researcher conducted one of the first empirical studies of the association of help-seeking behavior with both perceived public stigma and people's own stigmatizing attitudes (personal stigma). There were three main findings: (a) Perceived public stigma was considerably higher than personal stigma; (b) personal stigma was higher among students with any of the following characteristics: male, younger, Asian, international, more religious, or from a poor family; and (c) personal stigma was significantly and negatively associated with measures of help seeking (perceived need and use of psychotropic medication, therapy, and nonclinical sources of support), whereas perceived stigma was not significantly associated with help seeking..

4) Social support and mental health among college students

Hefner,J.E.(2009)

The aim of this study was to examine social support and mental health among college students. Total sample consisted of 1378 students in this research. The result reveals that students with characteristics differing from most other students, such as minority race or ethnicity, international status, and low socioeconomic status, are at greater risk of social isolation. In addition, the researcher found that students with lower quality social support were more likely to experience mental health problems, including a six fold risk of depressive symptoms relative to students with high quality social support. These results may help administrators and health providers to identify more effectively the population of students at high risk for mental illness and develop effective interventions to address this significant and growing public health issue.

5) Mental Health Services: Use and Disparity among Diverse College Students

B.H.Rosenthal(2008)

Objective: In this experimental study, the authors examined (1) actual use of counseling for emotional problems and (2) the assumptions that ethnicity, sex, social class, and psychological distress are associated with disparities in use of counseling.

Participants: There were 1,773 diverse undergraduate students from urban university.

Methods: The researcher use self-administered questionnaires between 1999 and 2005 to collect data; they used a cross-sectional correlation research design and analysis of variance statistical procedures.

Results: The level of students using counseling (10%) was similar to the estimation of the national college sample. Students reporting higher levels of Emergency use more counseling; however, more than three students who reported clinically critical crisis levels did not get the consultation

Conclusions: The researcher observed no disparities in use of mental health services in terms of sex, ethnicity, and socioeconomic status.

6) Mental health and stress among government and private B.ed college students

Janani Jalpa.A(2016)

Purpose: The purpose of the present study to find out mental health and stress among government and private B.Ed College students.

Methods: Total sample consisted of 120 B.Ed students, whom 60 were government B.Ed students and 60 were private B.ed students. The research tool for Mental Health was developed by Dr.D.J.Bhatt and Gita R.Gida and Life stress scale was developed by Agrawal and Naidu was used in this research. Here t-test and r was applied to check the significance difference and correlation between government and private B.Ed students.

Conclusion: The result revealed that significance difference in mental health and stress with respect to government and private B.Ed students, while the correlation between mental health and stress reveals 0.79, its very high positive correlation.

7) Cyber Disorders: The Mental Health Concern for the New Millennium

Kimberly Young (2009)

Anecdotal proof has recommended that mental health practitioners' statement improved caseloads of clients whose prime complaint involves the Internet. Though, little is recognized about the frequency, related behaviors, attitudes of practitioners, and interventions involved associated to this comparatively new incident. Therefore, this research surveyed therapists who have treated patients anguish from cyber-related troubles to gather such outcome information. Participants reported a normal caseload of 9 patients who accepted as Internet-addicted, with a range between 2 and 50 patients treated within the one year. Treatment strategies include cognitive behavioral behavior, sexually transmitted medicine, marital and family therapy, social skills training and medicinal interventions. Patients believe that efforts were made to support groups and recovery programs. Finally, on the base of the findings, this study reveals the impact of cyber disorders on future research, treatment, and public policy.

8) The Impact of Internet Addiction on Students' Mental Health in Technical and Vocational Colleges in Alborg Province

Ramezan J.K. & et.al (2013)

Uses of the Internet and its appeal in recent years have led to the appearance of a phenomenon known as "Internet addiction ". Internet itself is a risk-free tool but wrong usage of net may lead to the risk of addiction which accordingly might result in disruptions in mental health and social relationships. Thus, the here aims of this research is at investigating the level to which the Internet addiction may have impacts on students' mental health in technical and vocational colleges in Alborg province. Tis research is run on the basis of explanatory relative research method. In this research 260 female respondents were selected by stratified random sampling. General Health Questionnaire (GHQ) and Young Internet addiction test were use in this research. Explanatory and Inferential statistics have been used to analyze data. In addition, the obtained results indicate that regarding the occurrence of addiction to the Internet 36.6% of the subjects were slightly addicted to the Internet; 55.3% of the subjects were respectively addicted to the Internet; 7.3% of the subjects were moderately addicted to the Internet and 0.6% of the subjects were severely addicted to the Internet.

9) The Psychometric Properties of the Internet Addiction Test on Mental Health

Laura W.T. (2004)

In studying this subject, a valid and reliable evaluation instrument is necessary. In her survey of Internet addiction, Young designed the Internet Addiction Test (IAT), which provides a basis for developments. The IAT has high face validity, but it has not been subjected to organize psychometric testing. This research sought to duplicate and enlarge Young's survey, and to examine the IAT more systematically. A questionnaire web page was created, which included 15 other questions about the demographic data of IAT and respondents and Internet use. Respondents were recruited through the Internet, compliant 86 valid responses (29 males and 57 females). Factor analysis of the IAT revealed six factors—salience, excessive use, neglecting work, anticipation, lack of control, and neglecting social life. These factors showed good internal reliability and concurrent validity, with salience being the most reliable. Younger and more recent users revealed more troubles, mostly regarding the neglect of work and social life. We predictable interactive Internet functions to be more addictive; however, this was not found to be so. Overall, the IAT is a valid and reliable instrument that may be used in further study on Internet addiction.

10) Mental health and Occupational stress of female Nurses

Chothani K.B. (2015)

Aim: To examine mental health and occupational stress of female Nurses

Method:

Methods: Total sample consisted of 120 nurses, whom 60 were nurses of government hospitals and 60 were nurses of private hospitals of Ahmedabad. The research tool for Mental Health was developed by Jagdish & Srivastva and Occupational stress Index was developed by Srivastva and Singh was used in this research. Here t-test was applied to check the significance difference between government and private hospital nurses.

Conclusion: The result revealed that significance difference in mental health and Occupational stress with respect to nurses of government hospitals and nurses of private hospitals, while the nurses of government hospital posses more occupational stress in comparison to private hospital nurses.

Chapter 03: Methodology

3.1 Introduction

Any research starts with curiosities and many questions about a give phenomenon or set of phenomena. This section brings out explicitly how the research work has been carried out and which population is considered for the study, what sampling methods were under taken for the study, how the independent variables are measured and how the data is collected for the research work. The process of collecting data and analyzed the result by standardized tools in this research.

3.2 Research Problem

"INTERNET ADDICTION AND MENTAL HEALTH AMONG THE STUDENTS OF ARTS, COMMERCE AND SCIENCE FACULTY"

3.3 Objectives

The prime objectives of the study are as under.

1. To explore significant different of faculty variables on internet addiction.
2. To explore significant different of sex variables on internet addiction.
3. To explore significant different of area variables on internet addiction.
4. To explore significant different of interaction between faculty and sex variables on internet addiction.
5. To explore check significant different of interaction between faculty and area variables on internet addiction.
6. To explore significant different of interaction between area and sex variables on internet addiction.
7. To explore significant different of interaction between faculty, sex and area variables on internet addiction.
8. To explore significant different of faculty variables on mental health.
9. To explore significant different of sex variables of mental health.
10. To explore significant different of area variables on mental health.
11. 11. To explore significant different of interaction between faculty and sex variables on mental health.
12. To explore significant different of interaction between area and sex variables on mental health.

13. To explore significant different of interaction between faculty and area variables on mental health.
14. To explore significant different of interaction between faculty, area and sex variables on
15. Mental Health.
16. To check the correlation between internet addiction and mental health.

3.4 Hypothesis

Hypothesis of present research are as under:

1. There is no significance difference of Internet addiction based on types of faculty variable.
2. There is no significance difference of Internet addiction based on types of sex variable.
3. There is no significance difference of Internet addiction based on types of area variable.
4. There is no significance difference of Internet Addiction based on Interaction for types of faculty and Sex variables.
5. There is no significance difference of Internet Addiction based on Interaction for types of faculty and area variables.
6. There is no significance difference of Internet Addiction based on Interaction for sex and area variables.
7. There is no significance difference of Internet Addiction based on Interaction for types of faculty, Sex and Area variables.
8. There is no significance difference of Mental Health based on types of faculty variables.
9. There is no significance difference of Mental Health based on Sex variables.
10. There is no significance difference of Mental Heath based on Area variables.
11. There is no significance difference of Mental Health based on Interaction for types of faculty and Sex variables.
12. There is no significance difference of Mental Health based on Interaction for types of faculty and Area variables.

13. There is no significance difference of Mental Health based on Interaction of Sex and Area variables.
14. There is no significance difference of Mental Health based on Interaction for types of faculty, Sex and Area variables.
15. There is no significance difference of Perception of reality a part of Mental Health based on types of faculty variables.
17. There is no significance difference of Perception of reality a part of Mental Health based on Sex variables.
18. There is no significance difference of Perception of reality a part of Mental Heath based on Area variables.
19. There is no significance difference of Perception of reality a part of Mental Health based on Interaction for types of faculty and Sex variables.
20. There is no significance difference of Perception of reality a part of Mental Health based on Interaction for types of faculty and Area variables.
21. There is no significance difference of Perception of reality a part of Mental Health based on Interaction of Sex and Area variables.
22. There is no significance difference of Perception of reality a part of Mental Health based on Interaction for types of faculty, Sex and Area variables.
23. There is no significance difference of Integration of personality a part of Mental Health based on types of faculty variables.
24. There is no significance difference of Integration of personality a part of Mental Health based on Sex variables.
25. There is no significance difference of Integration of personality a part of Mental Heath based on Area variables.
26. There is no significance difference of Integration of personality a part of Mental Health based on Interaction for types of faculty and Sex variables.
27. There is no significance difference of Integration of personality a part of Mental Health based on Interaction for types of faculty and Area variables.
28. There is no significance difference of Integration of personality a part of Mental Health based on Interaction of Sex and Area variables.

29. There is no significance difference of Integration of personality a part of Mental Health based on Interaction for types of faculty, Sex and Area variables.
30. There is no significance difference of Positive self evolution a part of Mental Health based on types of faculty variables.
31. There is no significance difference of Positive self evolution a part of Mental Health based on Sex variables.
32. There is no significance difference of Positive self evolution a part of Mental Heath based on Area variables.
33. There is no significance difference of Positive self evolution a part of Mental Health based on Interaction for types of faculty and Sex variables.
34. There is no significance difference of Positive self evolution a part of Mental Health based on Interaction for types of faculty and Area variables.
35. There is no significance difference of Positive self evolution a part of Mental Health based on Interaction of Sex and Area variables.
36. There is no significance difference of Positive self evolution a part of Mental Health based on Interaction for types of faculty, Sex and Area variables.
37. There is no significance difference of Group oriented attitudes a part of Mental Health based on types of faculty variables.
38. There is no significance difference of Group oriented attitudes a part of Mental Health based on Sex variables.
39. There is no significance difference of Group oriented attitudes a part of Mental Heath based on Area variables.
40. There is no significance difference of Group oriented attitudes a part of Mental Health based on Interaction for types of faculty and Sex variables.
41. There is no significance difference of Group oriented attitudes a part of Mental Health based on Interaction for types of faculty and Area variables.
42. There is no significance difference of Group oriented attitudes a part of Mental Health based on Interaction for types of Sex and Area variables.
43. There is no significance difference of Group oriented attitudes a part of Mental Health based on Interaction for types of faculty, Sex and Area variables.

44. There is no significance difference of Environmental Mastery a part of Mental Health based on types of faculty variables.
45. There is no significance difference of Environmental Mastery a part of Mental Health based on Sex variables.
46. There is no significance difference of Environmental Mastery a part of Mental Heath based on Area variables.
47. There is no significance difference of Environmental Mastery a part of Mental Health based on Interaction for types of faculty and Sex variables.
48. There is no significance difference of Environmental Mastery a part of Mental Health based on Interaction for types of faculty and Area variables.
49. There is no significance difference of Environmental Mastery a part of Mental Health based on Interaction of Sex and Area variables.
50. There is no significance difference of Environmental Mastery a part of Mental Health based on Interaction for types of faculty, Sex and Area variables.
51. There is no correlation between Internet Addiction and Mental Health.
52. There is no significance mean difference between joint family and nuclear family on Internet addiction.
53. There is no significance mean difference between joint family and nuclear family on mental health

3.5 Research Variables

The following Research Variables are selected on the basis of the study which is as follow under,

3.5.1 Independent Variables

In present research total three independent variables are as under

A) Type of faculty: A1 = Arts A2= Commerce A3= Science

B) Sex: B1= Male B2= Female

C) Area: C1= Rural C2= Urban

3.5.2 Dependent variables

A total score of Internet Addiction and Mental Health are relying on Questionnaires.

1) Internet Addiction score

2) Mental Health score

3.6 Research Sample

The respondent of present study shall be **720 subjects**; data will collect from different area like Ahmadabad and Gandhinagar. The total sample is **720 students. 240 Arts, 240 Commerce and 240 Science** students are there. In subject of 240 out of which **120 are male** and **120 are female** student. In subject of **120** out of which **60 are from Urban** and **60 are from rural areas**.

3.7 The Research Plan

- **The research plan** for this study is **3x2x2 factorial design.** The respondent of present study shall be **720 subjects.**
- **A= faculty A1= Arts A2= Commerce , A3= Science**
- **B= Sex B1=Male B2=Female**
- **C= Area C1= Urban C2= Rural**

3.7.1 Research design:

The research design for this study is **3x2x2 factorial design,** as mentioned below

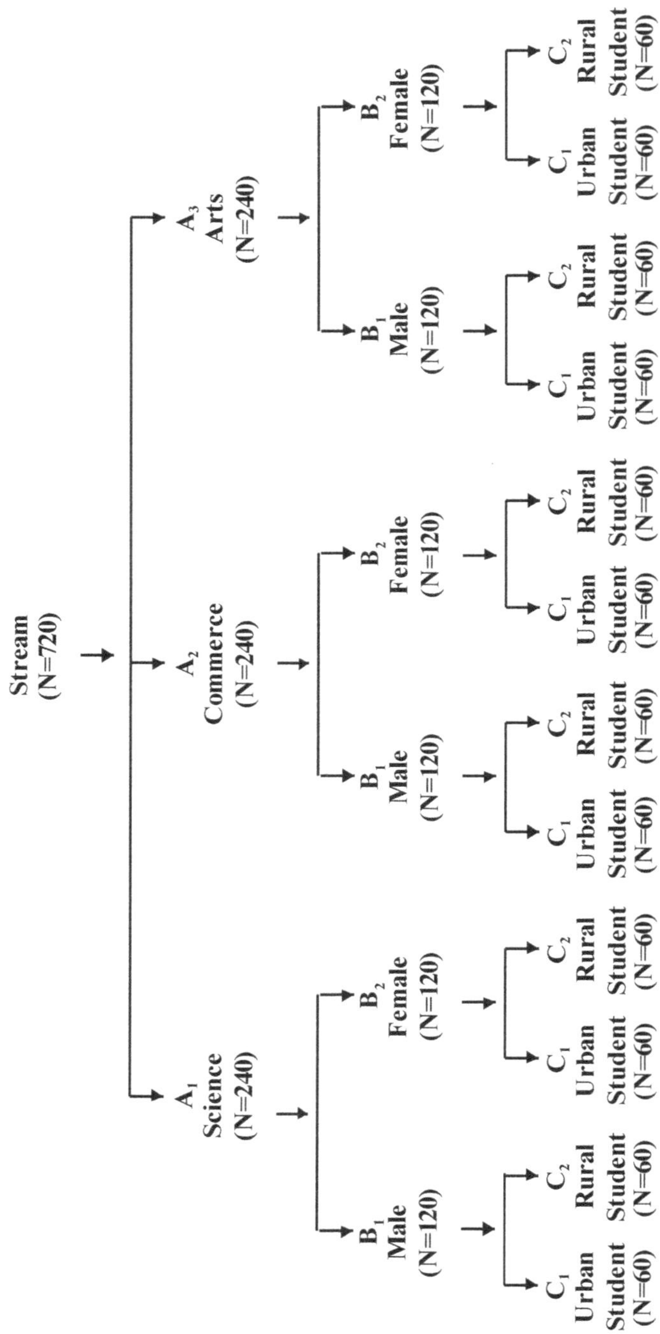
Stream (N=720)
A1 Science (N=240)
A2 Commerce (N=240)
A3 Arts (N=240)
B1 Male (N=120)
B2 Female (N=120)
B1 Male (N=120)
B2 Female (N=120)
B1 Male (N=120)
B2 Female (N=120)
C1 Urban Student (N=60)
C2 Rural Student (N=60)
C1 Urban Student (N=60)
C2 Rural Student (N=60)
C1 Urban Student (N=60)
C2 Rural Student (N=60)
C1 Urban Student (N=60)
C2 Rural Student (N=60)
C1 Urban Student (N=60)
C2 Rural Student (N=60)
C1 Urban Student (N=60)
C2 Rural Student (N=60)

3.8 Research Tools

In this research personal data is preparing to collect some personal data for the students.

3.8.1 Personal data sheet

In this research personal data sheet is preparing by researcher to collect some personal information such as Type of Faculty, Sex, Area, How many hours uses of Internet, Age, Income , Doing Part time job or Not etc.

3.8.2 Internet addiction test

Internet addiction test was developed by Kimbal Young. In this research use the Guajarati adaption of this test by Mittal Vekariya. It consists of 20 items that measures mind, moderate and severe level of internet addiction. This scale was depended on five-point Likert scale. The score of this test was classified into normal users (score <20), mild (score 20-49), moderate (score 50-79) and severe (score >79) internet addiction, so it's a very clear about the norms made by Kimbal Young in original scale. The maximum score on Internet addiction test is 100 and minimum score is 20. The reality and reliability and validity of this test are high.

3.8.3 Mental health Questionnaire

In this research Mental Health Questionnaire was developed by Dr. D.J Bhatt and Geeta R.Gida will use. It consists of 40 items. It is three point scale like as agree, disagree and neutral. When sentence is positive then scoring is agree=3, disagree=2 and neutral=1, if sentence is negative the scoring is agree=2, disagree=3and neutral=1.Maximun score is 120 and minimum score is 40. There is a five parts of Mental Health questionnaire like as Perception of reality, Integration of personality, Positive self evolution, Group Oriented attitudes and Environmental Mastery.

The item numbers 1,6,11,16,21,26,31,36 are measure to Perception of reality, the item numbers of 2,7,12,17,22,27,32,37 are measure Integration of personality, The item numbers of 3,8,13,18,23,28,33,38 are measure Positive self evolution, the item numbers of 4,9,14,19,24,29,34,39 are measure Group Oriented Attitudes and the items number of 5,10,15,20,25,30,35,40 are measure Environmental Mastery. The item numbers of 1,3,9,14,19,20,22,24,25,26,28,33,35,37and38 are negative sentences. The reliability of Mental Health Questionnaire checked by three methods, Split half reliability was 0.94, Test-retest reliability was 0.87 and parallel forms reliability was 0.80. The content validity of this questionnaire was 0.63.

3.9 Statistical frame work for the study

The respondent of present study shall be **720 subject** randomly selected from different area of Ahmadabad and Gandhinagar Dist. in Gujarat state. So collect the data as **3x2x2** factorial design, after than data collection to choose some statistical techniques for interpretation of the result. The **"F"** test will apply to examine significant difference of main and internal effect of gender, educational stream and area.

3.9.1 F-Test

The F-test is also known as the Variance (ANOVA). This test was developed by Fisher. This exam is not just a statistical method; this is an approach that can be used to evaluate the ANOVA F test, whether any therapy is average or lesser than others, which responds equally to all indivisible reactions. This is an example of the "omnipresent" exam, which means that one test is done. Alternatively, we can do the same testing as treatment (for example, in the example of a medical test with four treatments)

The benefits of ANOVA are that we do not have to fix the treatment type before, and we do not have to compile multiple comparisons. The disadvantage of ANOVA is that if we reject the null hypothesis we cannot know who is different from the second treatment, we can tell the F-level we set the difference in the difference with α is an important difference. The formula for the one-way ANOVA F-test statistic is F= Explained variance / UN Explained variance or

F= between group variability/ within group variability

3.9.2 Least significant difference (L.S.D.)

Fisher's LSD treatment is a method of comparing the group, which means that the null nature of the same equipment has been rejected using ANOVA,F-test. If F-test fails to deny defiance, it should not be used. Note that LSD has more power than other post-hoc comparison methods.

3.9.3 t-test

A simple test of a t-test is a statistical test that is associated with an unknown standard deviation through the general population; Sample used to split standard deviation of samples of the number of persons in the average and sample number as a result of the population divided by the equivalent variable of the variable used in the sample.

3.9.4 Correlation(r)

Correlation very useful statistics are Pearson product-moment correlation coefficient, or "Pearson's correlation." They are obtained by dividing the two variables by standard deviation; Karl Pearson develops coefficients with a similar but slightly different view by Francis Galton. A relation is a single number that describes the degree of relation between the two variables. Correlation coefficient is a numerical value which indicates the degree and direction of two variables. Coefficient shows the correct positive affinity of +1.00 values, 0.00 does not show any relation and -1.00 shows the perfect negative or inverse relationship between the two variables

3.10 The Data collection

This section brings out the various organizations in which the study was undertaken and under which guidance the study was authorized. Hemchandracharya North Gujarat University, Dept of Psychology, Patan authenticated the research work and under the guidance of Dr. Chhayaben Suchak. Here the Research practice and Data collection for various college students, under the guidance was undertaken with the help of Dr.Chhayaben Suchak and various principals and professor.

The respondents of present study shall be 720 Subjects, total 980 data fill up from different areas & hospitals, in which randomly selected 720 data from different areas (e.g. Gandhinagar, Ahemdabad, Visnagar etc.) & different colleges from Gujarat state. The group was randomly selected by administering the testing inventories. The library of Hemchandracharya University, The library of Gujarat University, the Library of Government Arts College, Gandhinagar have largely benefited in collection. So the process of the data collection as follows;

The aim of present study was compare the Internet Addiction and Mental Health among the students of Arts, Commerce and Science faculty. For this purpose the following test tools were considered with their reliability, validity and objectivity mentioned in their respective manuals. There are two (02) Inventories used in this research. Here used to collect the data for Internet Addiction test was developed by Kimbal Young and in regional language translated and standardized by Mittal Vekariya used in this research.

Used to collect the data for Mental Health, the questionnaire for Mental Health was developed by D.J.Bhatt and Gita R.Gida used in this research. So here the respondents of present study shall be 720 Subjects, randomly selected from different colleges and areas of Ahmedabad, Gandhinagar and Visnagar of Gujarat state. The total sample consisting of 720 Subjects out which 240 are Arts students, 240 are Commerece students and 240 are Science students. In subjects of 240 out of which 120 are male and 120 are female. In subjects of 120 out of which 60 are rural students and 60 are urban students were taken for this study.

Chapter 04: Result, Discussion and Interpretation

4.1 Introduction

This section brings out the analysis technique used by the investigator and the interpretation of the results obtained. This section brings out the Suggestion for improvement for further research work in the similar field. In the previous chapter the sample, design, hypothesis, different tool are used, method of administration of the tool and the statistical analysis were described. In every research analysis and interpretation of data is the most important task. The result of the present study will be presented, interpreted and discussed in this chapter .In order to test various hypotheses put forward the following analysis was carried out.

In this study to find out main and interaction effects of the three independent variables F-test was applied. LSD test was also computed to find out significant differences for interacting subgroups. To find out correlation between two variables used Karl Pearson`s correlation methods.

4.2 Percentages Tabulations of Research Data

The aim of present research was **'INTERNET ADDICTION AND MENTAL HEALTH AMONG THE STUDENTS OF ARTS, COMMERCE AND SCIENCE FACULTY'** so; here according to sample has been selected from **3x2x2 research design**. Hence it could be show the Distribution of different samples as under;

4.2.1 The percentage wise distribution for total research sample

The respondents of present study shall be **720** samples, which **240** are Arts faculty student, **240** are commerce faculty students and **240** are science faculty students.

Table 4.2.1

The percentage wise distribution for Types of faculty variables

No.	Name of Variables	N	Percentage
1	Arts faculty students	240	33.33%
2	Commerce faculty students	240	33.33%
3	Science faculty students	240	33.33%
	Total	**700**	**100%**

The respondents of present study shall be 720 samples, which 240 are from Arts faculty students,240 are from Commerce faculty students and rest 240 are from Science faculty students. So we can said that the respondents of the present study shall be 720 samples, out of which 33.33%samples from Arts faculty students,33.33%samples from Commerce faculty students and rest 33.33% samples from Science faculty students.

4.2.2 The percentage wise distribution for sex variables

The respondents of present study shall be **720** samples, which **360** are male students and **360** are female students. These despondences were from different colleges.

Table 4.2.2
The percentage wise distribution for sex variables

No.	Variables (sex)	N	Percentage
1	Male students	360	50.00%
2	Female students	360	50.00%
3	Total	**720**	**100%**

The respondents of present study shall be 720 samples, which 360 are male students and 360 are female students. In present study 50% samples were male students and rest 50% were female students.

4.2.3 The percentage wise distribution for Area variable

Table 4.2.3
The percentage wise distribution for Area variables

No.	Variables (Area)	N	Percentage
1	Rural	360	50.00%
2	Urban	360	50.00%
3	Total	**720**	**100%**

The respondent for the present study shall be 720 samples, which 360 are from Rural area and 360 are from Urban area. So we can said that the respondent of the present study shall be 720 students, out of which 50% samples from Rural area and rest 50% samples from Urban area.

4.3. The Respondents socio personal variables and their 3x2x2 factorial design for Internet addiction

While the data collection was completed then F test ANOVAs, t-test, L.S.D. and correlation applied to check significance difference between students of Arts faculty, Commerce faculty and Science faculty. So here first of all presented the mean and S.D. score for independent variables on Internet Addiction and after them shows the result for ANOVAs, t-test, L.S.D. and correlations between the students of Arts faculty, Commerce faculty and Science faculty. So all results and result discussion are as under;

Table 4.3.1
The Mean score and Standard Deviation score for Independent variables on Internet Addiction

Variables	A1(Arts faculty)		A2(Commerce faculty)		A3(Science faculty)	
	B1(male students)	B2(female students)	B1(male students)	B2(female students)	B1(male students)	B2(female students)
C1 (Rural area)	∑X=2666 MX=44.43 S.D.=15.12 N=60	∑X=3031 MX=50.52 S.D.=13.40 N=60	∑X=2702 MX=45.03 S.D.=13.82 N=60	∑X=2265 MX=37.75 S.D.=12.70 N=60	∑X=2790 MX=46.50 S.D.=13.02 N=60	∑X=2616 MX=43.6 S.D.=15.25 N=60
C2 (Urban area)	∑X=2826 MX=47.1 S.D.=18.83 N=60	∑X=2443 MX=40.72 S.D.=14.47 N=60	∑X=2858 MX=38.17 S.D.=14.33 N=60	∑X=2271 MX=37.85 S.D.=11.61 N=60	∑X=2923 MX=48.72 S.D.=15.34 N=60	∑X=2803 MX=46.72 S.D.=17.51 N=60

It could be seen from the table No.**4.3.1** the mean score and S.D. score for Independent variables on Internet addiction. The highest mean score was 50.52 of rural female from Arts faculty students and the lowest mean score was 37.75 of rural female from Commerce faculty students.

Table No.4.3.2

F calculation for Internet Addiction (3x2x2 factorial designed)

Sources of variance	Sum of square	d.f.	Mean square	F	Significanc e level
Ass (Types of faculty)	2597.27	2	1298.63	5.96	0.01
Bss (Sex)	5841.63	1	5841.63	26.82	0.01
Css (Area)	15.72	1	15.72	0.072	N.S.
ABss	998.02	2	466.01	2.29	N.S.
ACss	1106.35	2	553.17	2.54	N.S.
BCss	37.45	1	37.45	0.172	N.S.
ABCss	56.72	2	28.36	0.13	N.S.
Wss	154228.23	708	217.84	-	-
Tss	164839.06	719	-	-	-

Significance levels df_1 0.05 = 3.85, 0.01= 6.66
df_2 0.05 = 3.00, 0.01= 4.62

From the table **No.4.3.2** it is clear that F value of types of faculty variables was **5.96**, which was significance at **0.01** levels. The F value of sex variables was **26.82**, which was significance at **0.01** levels. The F value of Area variables was **0.072**, which was not significance at **0.05** levels. The F value of Interaction to Types of faculty and Sex variables was **2.29**, which was not significance at **0.05** levels. The F value of Interaction to types of faculty and Area variables was **2.54**, which was not significance at **0.05** levels.

The F value of Interaction to Sex and Area variables was **0.172**, which was not significance at **0.05** levels. The F value of Interaction to types of faculty, Sex and Area variables was **0.13**.

Ho_1: There is no significance difference of Internet addiction based on types of faculty variable.

Table No. 4.3.3
The mean and F value for Types of faculty variable on Internet addiction

No.	Variables	N	Mean	F	Sig.
1	Arts faculty students (A_1)	240	45.71	**5.96**	**0.01**
2	Commerce faculty students(A_2)	240	42.07		
3	Science faculty students(A3)	240	46.36		

Significance levels df_2 = 0.05=3.00 / 0.01=4.63

Table No 4.3.4
L.S.D. for Types of faculty variables on Internet addiction

No.	Variables	N	Mean diff.	Sig.
1	Arts faculty students(A_1) vs. Commerce faculty students(A_2)	240	**3.64**	**0.01**
2	Arts faculty students(A_1) vs. Science faculty students(A_3)	240	**0.65**	**N.S.**
3	Commerce faculty students(A_2) vs. Science faculty students(A_3)	240	**4.29**	**0.01**

Significance levels for L.S.D. = 0.05=2.64 / 0.01=3.47

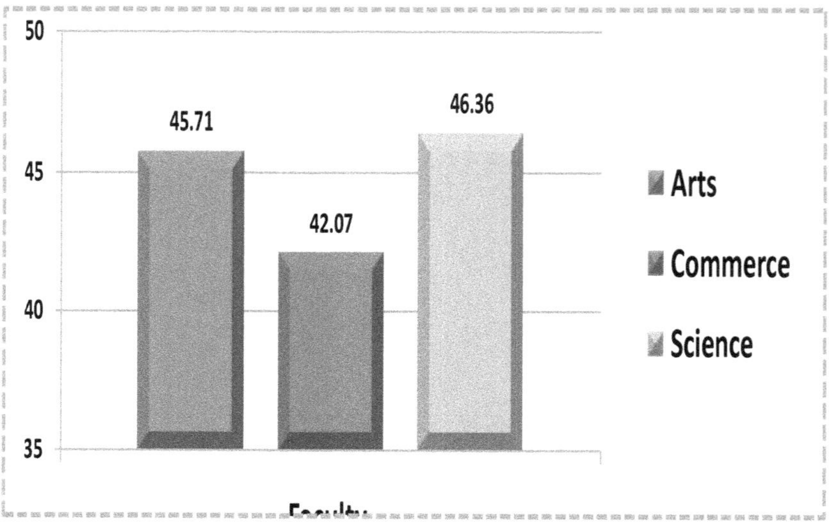

Figure.No.01
Bar chart of mean score of faculty on Internet addiction

The table No.**4.3.3** indicated that the mean for Arts faculty students were **45.71**, the mean for Commerce faculty students was **42.07** the mean for Science faculty students were **46.36.** The F value for Types of faculty variables was **5.96**, which was significance at **0.01** levels. So it could be seen the result and said that the mean score of Science faculty students was higher than other faculties on Internet addiction. Hence, the **Ho_1** was rejected and it could be said that there was significant mean difference between Types of faculty & their Internet Addiction. It could be seen from table No. **4.3.4** and figure no.01it shown L.S.D. for Types of faculty variables on Internet Addiction. The mean different between Arts faculty students and Commerce faculty students on Internet addiction was **3.64** which was Significance at **0.05** levels.

Thus we concluded that the students of Arts faculty are more Internet addicted than students of Commerce faculty. The mean different between Arts faculty students and Science faculty students on Internet addiction were **0.65** which was not significance at 0.05 levels. The mean different between Commerce faculty students and Science faculty students on Internet addiction were **4.29**.that which was Significance at **0.01** levels. Thus it concluded that the students of Arts faculty are more Internet addicted than students of Commerce faculty.

Ho_2: There is no significance difference of Internet addiction based on Sex variables.

Table No 4.3.5

The mean score and F value for Sex variables on Internet addiction

No.	Variables(Sex)	N	Mean	F	Sig.
1	Male students (B_1)	360	**47.55**	**26.82**	**0.01**
2	Female students (B_2)	360	**41.88**		

Significance levels dfl =0.05=3.85 / 0.01=6.66

Table No 4.3.6

L.S.D. for Types of Sex variables on Internet addiction

No.	Variables(Sex)	N	Mean diff.	Sig.
1	Male students (B_1)	360	**5.67**	**0.01**
2	Female students (B_2)	360		

Significance levels for L.S.D. =0.05=2.15 / 0.01=2.83

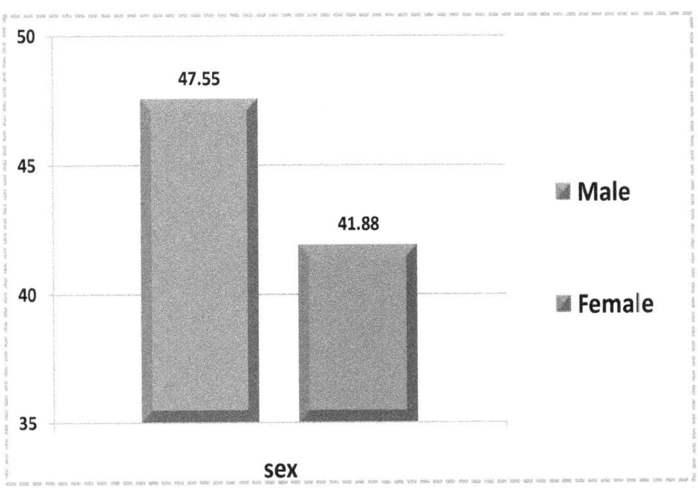

Figure No.2

Bar chart of mean score of sex variables on Internet addiction

From the table No. **4.3.5** it is observed that the mean for male students was **47.55** and the mean for Female students was **41.88**. The F value for sex variables was **26.82,** which was significance at **0.01** levels. Hence, the **Ho_2** was rejected and it could be said that there was significant mean difference between types of sex & their Internet Addiction score. So it observed the result and said that the male students are more Internet addicted than female students. Hence we concluded that Internet Addiction was very affected factor for male students. It could be seen from the table No. **4.3.6** and figure **No.02** the L.S.D. for Types of Sex variables on Internet Addiction that the mean different between Male and Female students on Internet Addiction was **5.67**, which was Significance at **0.01** levels. Thus it concluded that the Male students are more Internet Addicted than Female students. Hence it concluded that Internet Addiction was very affected factor for Male students.

Ho_3: There is no significance difference of Internet Addiction based on Area variables.

Table No 4.3.7

The mean score and F value for Area variables on Internet Addiction

No.	Variables(Area)	N	Mean	F	Sig.
1	Rural students (c_1)	360	**44.55**	**0.07**	**N.S.**
2	Urban students (c_2)	360	**44.88**		

Significance levels dfl =0.05=3.85 / 0.01=6.66

Table No 4.3.8

L.S.D. for Types of Area variables on Internet Addiction

No.	Variables(Area)	N	Mean diff.	Sig.
1	Rural students (c_1)	360	**0.33**	**N.S.**
2	Urban students (c_2)	360		

Significance levels for L.S.D. =0.05=2.15 / 0.01=2.83

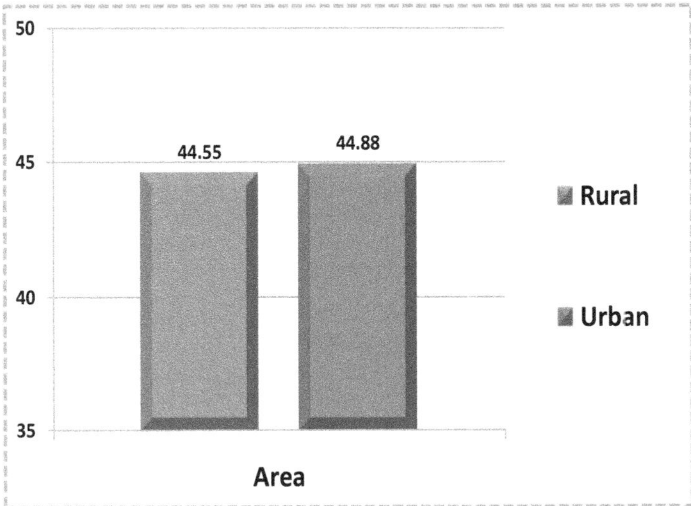

Figure No.3
Bar chart of mean score of area variable on Internet addiction

It could be seen from table No. **4.3.7** that the mean for rural students was **44.55** and the mean for Urban students was **44.88**. The F value for Area variables was **0.07**, which was not significant at **0.05** levels. Hence, the **Ho₃** was not rejected and it could be said that there was not significant mean difference between Types of area & their Internet Addiction score. So it saw the result and said that the urban students are more Internet Addicted than rural students. Hence it could be concluded that Internet Addiction is very affected factor for urban students.

From the table No. **4.3.8** and figure No.03 it is clear that the L.S.D. for types of area variables on Internet Addiction that the mean different between Rural students and Urban students on Internet Addiction was **0.33**, which was not Significance at **0.05** levels. Thus it concluded that the urban students are more Internet Addicted than rural students. Hence it could be conclude that Internet Addiction was very affected factor for urban students. Here, **Ho₃** is not rejected at 0.05 significant levels.

Ho_4: There is no significance difference of Internet Addiction based on Interaction for types of faculty and Sex variables.

Table No 4.3.9
Interaction F for types of faculty and Sex variables on Internet Addiction

Variables	A_1 (Arts students)	A_2 (commerce students)	A_3 (Science students)	F	Sig.
B_1 (Male students)	**48.80**	**46.33**	**47.61**	**2.29**	**N.S.**
B_2 (Female students)	**42.58**	**37.8**	**45.16**		

Significance levels df2 =0.05=3.00 / 0.01=4.63

Table No 4.3.10
A L.S.D. Table for Interaction of Types of faculty and Sex variables on Internet Addiction

Sr.N0.	Pairs	Mean Diff.	Significance
1	A_1B_1 vs. A_1B_2	6.22	0.01
2	A_1B_1 vs. A_2B_1	2.47	N.S.
3	A_1B_1 vs. A_2B_2	11.00	0.01
4	A_1B_1 vs.A_3B_1	1.19	N.S.
5	A_1B_1 vs.A_3B_2	3.16	0.05
6	A_1B_2 vs. A_2B_1	3.75	0.01
7	A_1B_2 vs. A_2B_2	4.78	0.01
8	A_1B_2 vs. A_3B_1	5.03	0.01
9	A_1B_2 vs.A_3B_2	2.58	N.S.
10	A_2B_1 vs.A_2B_2	8.53	0.01
11	A_2B_1 vs.A_3B_1	1.28	N.S.
12	A_2B_1 vs.A_3B_2	1.17	N.S.
13	A_2B_2 vs.A_3B_1	9.81	0.01
14	A_2B_2 vs.A_3B_2	7.36	0.01
15	A_3B_1 vs.A_3B_2	2.45	N.S.

Sig. levels for L.S.D. 0.05=3.74 / 0.01=4.89

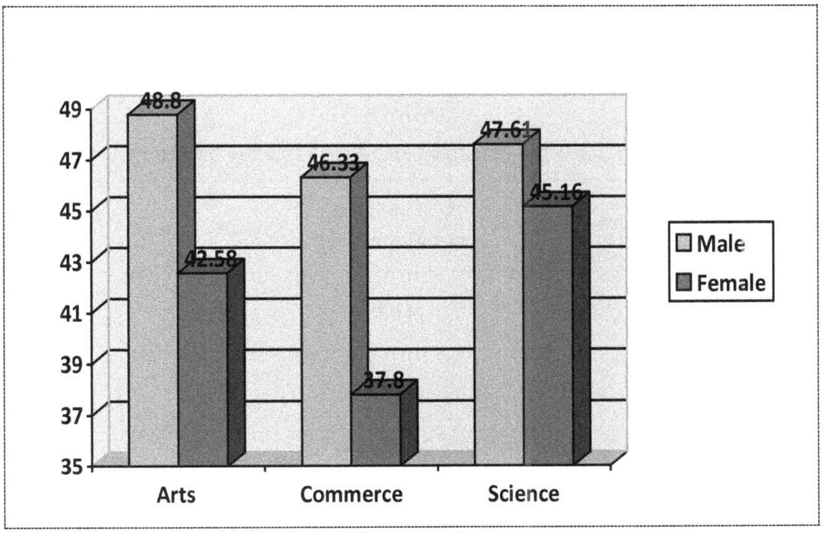

Figure No.04

Bar chart of interaction of Faculty and Sex variables on Internet addiction

It could be seen from the table No.**4.3.9** that the Interaction F for Types of faculty and Sex variables on Internet Addiction F value was **2.29**, which was not significance at **0.05** levels. Hence, the $\mathbf{Ho_5}$ was not rejected and it could be said that there was not significant mean difference between Types of faculty and sex variables & their Internet Addiction score. The table no.**4.3.10** and figure **No.04** point out the L.S.D. for interaction of types of faculty and sex variables on Internet Addiction. It could be seen the result and said that most of the pairs are significance at 0.05 or 0.01 levels. It could also said that the highest mean score **48.80** was Arts male students. So It could be said that Arts male students are more Internet Addicted students. The highest mean difference between A_1B_1 vs. A_2B_2 (Arts male students Vs. Commerce female students) was **11.00**, so the result said that it was big difference. The lowest mean difference between A_2B_1 vs. A_3B_2 (Commerce male students Vs. Science female students) was **1.17** on Internet Addiction. Hence, it could be seen all the result and concluded that either all variables (faculties and sex) are affected on Internet Addiction or Internet Addiction was affected them.

H_{05}: There is no significance difference of Internet Addiction based on Interaction for types of faculty and Area variables.

Table No 4.3.11

Interaction F for types of faculty and Area variables on Internet Addiction

Variables	A_1 (Arts faculty students)	A_2 (Commerce faculty students)	A_3 (Science faculty students)	F	Sig.
C_1 (Rural)	**47.48**	**41.39**	**45.05**	**2.54**	**N.S.**
C_2 (Urban)	**43.91**	**42.74**	**47.72**		

Significance levels df2 =0.05=3.00 /0.01=4.63

Table No 4.3.12

A L.S.D. Table for Interaction of Types of faculty and Area variables on Internet Addiction

Sr.N0.	Pairs	Mean Diff.	Significance
1	A_1C_1 vs. A_1C_2	3.57	0.01
2	A_1C_1 vs. A_2C_1	6.09	0.01
3	A_1C_1 vs. A_2C_2	4.74	0.01
4	A_1C_1 vs.A_3C_1	2.43	N.S.
5	A_1C_1 vs.A_3C_2	0.24	N.S.
6	A_1C_2 vs. A_2C_1	2.52	N.S.
7	A_1C_2 vs. A_2C_2	1.17	N.S.
8	A_1C_2 vs. A_3C_1	1.14	N.S.
9	A_1C_2 vs.A_3C_2	3.81	0.01
10	A_2C_1 vs.A_2C_2	1.35	N.S.
11	A_2C_1 vs.A_3C_1	3.66	0.01
12	A_2C_1 vs.A_3C_2	6.33	0.01
13	A_2C_2 vs.A_3C_1	2.31	N.S.
14	A_2C_2 vs.A_3C_2	4.98	0.01
15	A_3C_1 vs.A_3C_2	2.67	0.05

Sig. levels for L.S.D. 0.05=3.75/ 0.01=4.89

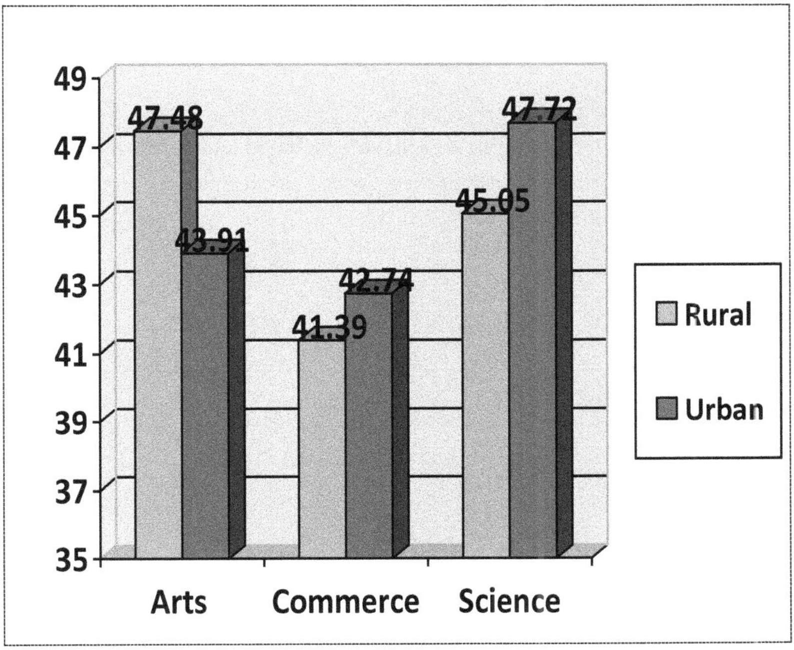

Figure No.05

Bar chart of interaction of Faculty and Area variables on Internet addiction

It is observed from the table No.**4.3.11** that the Interaction F for Types of faculty and Area variables on Internet Addiction F value was **2.54**, which was not significance at **0.05** levels. Hence, the **Ho_5** was not rejected and it could be said that there was significant mean difference between Types of faculty and area variables & their Internet Addiction score. The table no.**4.3.12** and figure **No.05** reveals L.S.D. for interaction between the types of faculty and area variables on Internet addiction. That it could be seen the result and said that the most of pairs significance at 0.05 or 0.01 levels. The result also said the highest mean difference between A_2C_1 vs.A_3C_2 (Commerce rural students Vs. Science urban students) was **6.33**,so it can said that it was big difference. The lowest mean difference between A_1C_1 vs.A_3C_2 (Arts rural students Vs. Science Urban students) was **0.24** on Internet Addiction.

Ho_6: There is no significance difference of Internet Addiction based on Interaction for Sex variables and Area variables.

Table No 4.3.13
Interaction F for Sex variables and Area variables on Internet Addiction

Variables	B_1 (Male students)	B_2 (Female students)	F	Sig.
Rural students (C_1)	47.35	41.93	**0.17**	**N.S.**
Urban students (C_2)	47.82	41.76		

Sig. levels df_2 =0.05=3.85 / 0.01=6.66

Table No 4.3.14
A L.S.D. Table for Interaction of Sex and Area variables on Internet Addiction

Sr.No.	Pairs	Mean Diff.	Significance
1	B_1C_1 vs. B_1C_2	0.47	N.S.
2	B_1C_1 vs. B_2C_1	5.42	0.01
3	B_1C_1 vs. B_2C_2	5.59	0.01
4	B_1C_2 vs.B_2C_1	5.89	0.01
5	B_1C_2 vs. B_2C_2	6.06	0..01
6	B_2C_1 vs. B_2C_2	0.17	N.S.

Sig. levels for L.S.D. 0.05=3.77/ 0.01=4.89

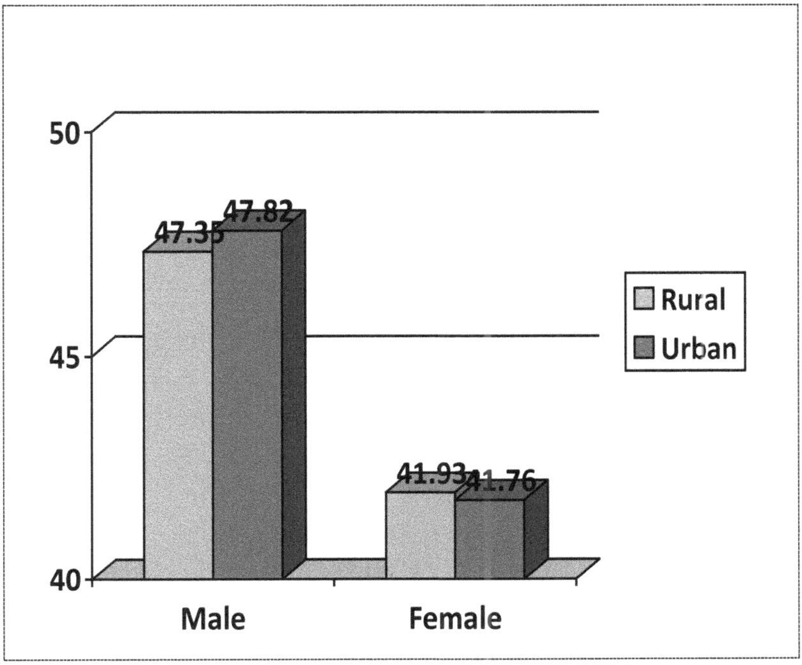

Figure No. 06
Bar chart of interaction between sex and area variables on Internet Addiction

It could be seen from the table No.**4.3.13** that the Interaction F for Sex variables and Area variables on Internet Addiction F value was **0.013**, which was not significance at **0.05** levels. Hence, the **Ho_6** was not rejected at 0.05 levels and it could be said that there was no significant mean difference between Sex variables and Area variables & their Internet Addiction score.

The table **4.3.14** and figure **No.06** indicated the L.S.D. for interaction between the Sex variables and Area variables on Internet addiction, that it seen the result and said that most of pairs are significance at 0.01 levels. It present highest mean difference between B_1C_2 vs. B_2C_1 (male urban students Vs. female rural students) was 6.06, so it could be said that it was big difference. The lowest mean difference score between B_2C_1 vs. B_2C_2 (female rural students vs. female urban students) was 0.17 on Internet addiction.

Ho_7: There is no significance difference of Internet Addiction based on Interaction for types of faculty, Sex and Area variables.

Table No 4.3.15

Interaction F for types of Faculty, Sex and Area variables on Internet Addiction

Variables	A_1 (Arts students)		A_2 (Commerce students)		A_3 (Science students)		F	Sign.
	B_1 male students	B_2 female students	B_1 male students	B_2 female students	B_1 male students	B_2 female students		
C_1	50.52	44.43	45.03	37.75	46.5	43.6	0.13	N.S.
C_2	47.1	40.72	47.63	37.85	48.72	46.72		

Significance levels df_1 =0.05=3.00 / 0.01=4.63

Table No 4.3.16

A L.S.D. Table for Interaction of Sex and Area variables on Internet Addiction

Sr.No.	Pairs	Mean Diff.	Significance
1	$A_1B_1C_1$ vs. $A_1B_1C_2$	3.42	N.S.
2	$A_1B_1C_1$ vs. $A_1B_2C_1$	6.09	0.05
3	$A_1B_1C_1$ vs. $A_1B_2C_2$	9.8	0.01
4	$A_1B_1C_1$ vs. $A_2B_1C_1$	5.49	0.05
5	$A_1B_1C_1$ vs. $A_2B_1C_2$	2.89	N.S.
6	$A_1B_1C_1$ vs. $A_2B_2C_1$	12.77	0.01
7	$A_1B_1C_1$ vs. $A_2B_2C_2$	12.67	0.01
8	$A_1B_1C_1$ vs. $A_3B_1C_1$	4.02	N.S.
9	$A_1B_1C_1$ vs. $A_3B_1C_2$	1.80	N.S.
10	$A_1B_1C_1$ vs. $A_3B_2C_1$	6.92	0.05
11	$A_1B_1C_1$ vs. $A_3B_2C_2$	3.80	N.S.
12	$A_1B_1C_2$ vs. $A_1B_2C_1$	2.67	N.S.
13	$A_1B_1C_2$ vs. $A_1B_2C_2$	6.38	0.05
14	$A_1B_1C_2$ vs. $A_2B_1C_1$	2.07	N.S.
15	$A_1B_1C_2$ vs. $A_2B_1C_2$	0.53	N.S.
16	$A_1B_1C_2$ vs. $A_2B_2C_1$	9.35	0.01
17	$A_1B_1C_2$ vs. $A_2B_2C_2$	9.25	0.01
18	$A_1B_1C_2$ vs. $A_3B_1C_1$	0.60	N.S.

19	$A_1B_1C_2$ vs. $A_3B_1C_2$	1.62	N.S
20	$A_1B_1C_2$ vs. $A_3B_2C_1$	3.50	N.S
21	$A_1B_1C_2$ vs. $A_3B_2C_2$	0.38	N.S
22	$A_1B_2C_1$ vs. $A_1B_2C_2$	3.71	N.S
23	$A_1B_2C_1$ vs. $A_2B_1C_1$	0.60	N.S
24	$A_1B_2C_1$ vs. $A_2B_1C_2$	3.20	N.S
25	$A_1B_2C_1$ vs. $A_2B_2C_1$	6.68	0.05
26	$A_1B_2C_1$ vs. $A_2B_2C_2$	6.85	0.05
27	$A_1B_2C_1$ vs. $A_3B_1C_1$	2.07	N.S.
28	$A_1B_2C_1$ vs. $A_3B_1C_2$	4.29	N.S.
29	$A_1B_2C_1$ vs. $A_3B_2C_1$	0.83	N.S.
30	$A_1B_2C_1$ vs. $A_3B_2C_2$	2.29	N.S.
31	$A_1B_2C_2$ vs. $A_2B_1C_1$	4.31	N.S.
32	$A_1B_2C_2$ vs. $A_2B_1C_2$	6.91	0.05
33	$A_1B_2C_2$ vs. $A_2B_2C_1$	2.97	N.S.
34	$A_1B_2C_2$ vs. $A_2B_2C_2$	2.87	N.S.
35	$A_1B_2C_2$ vs. $A_3B_1C_1$	5.78	0.05
36	$A_1B_2C_2$ vs. $A_3B_1C_2$	8.00	0.01
37	$A_1B_2C_2$ vs. $A_3B_2C_1$	2.88	N.S.
38	$A_1B_2C_2$ vs. $A_3B_2C_2$	6.00	0.05
39	$A_2B_1C_1$ vs. $A_2B_1C_2$	2.60	N.S.
40	$A_2B_1C_1$ vs. $A_2B_2C_1$	7.28	0.01
41	$A_2B_1C_1$ vs. $A_2B_2C_2$	7.18	0.01
42	$A_2B_1C_1$ vs. $A_3B_1C_1$	1.47	N.S.
43	$A_2B_1C_1$ vs. $A_3B_1C_2$	3.69	N.S.
44	$A_2B_1C_1$ vs. $A_3B_2C_1$	1.43	N.S.
45	$A_2B_1C_1$ vs. $A_3B_2C_2$	1.69	N.S.
46	$A_2B_1C_2$ vs. $A_2B_2C_1$	9.88	0.01
47	$A_2B_1C_2$ vs. $A_2B_2C_2$	9.78	0.01
48	$A_2B_1C_2$ vs. $A_3B_1C_1$	1.13	N.S.
49	$A_2B_1C_2$ vs. $A_3B_1C_2$	1.09	N.S.
50	$A_2B_1C_2$ vs. $A_3B_2C_1$	4.03	N.S.
51	$A_2B_1C_2$ vs. $A_3B_2C_2$	0.91	N.S.

52	$A_2B_2C_1$ vs. $A_2B_2C_2$	0.10	N.S.
53	$A_2B_2C_1$ vs. $A_3B_1C_1$	8.75	0.01
54	$A_2B_2C_1$ vs. $A_3B_1C_2$	10.97	0.01
55	$A_2B_2C_1$ vs. $A_3B_2C_1$	5.85	0.05
56	$A_2B_2C_1$ vs. $A_3B_2C_2$	8.97	0.01
57	$A_2B_2C_2$ vs. $A_3B_1C_1$	8.65	0.01
58	$A_2B_2C_2$ vs. $A_3B_1C_2$	10.87	0.01
59	$A_2B_2C_2$ vs. $A_3B_2C_1$	5.75	0.05
60	$A_2B_2C_2$ vs. $A_3B_2C_2$	8.87	0.01
61	$A_3B_1C_1$ vs. $A_3B_1C_2$	2.22	N.S.
62	$A_3B_1C_1$ vs. $A_3B_2C_1$	2.90	N.S.
63	$A_3B_1C_1$ vs. $A_3B_2C_2$	0.22	N.S.
64	$A_3B_1C_2$ vs. $A_3B_2C_1$	5.12	N.S.
65	$A_3B_1C_2$vs. $A_3B_2C_2$	2.00	N.S.
66	$A_3B_2C_1$ vs. $A_3B_2C_2$	3.12	N.S.

Sig. levels for L.S.D. 0.05=5.27/ 0.01=6.89

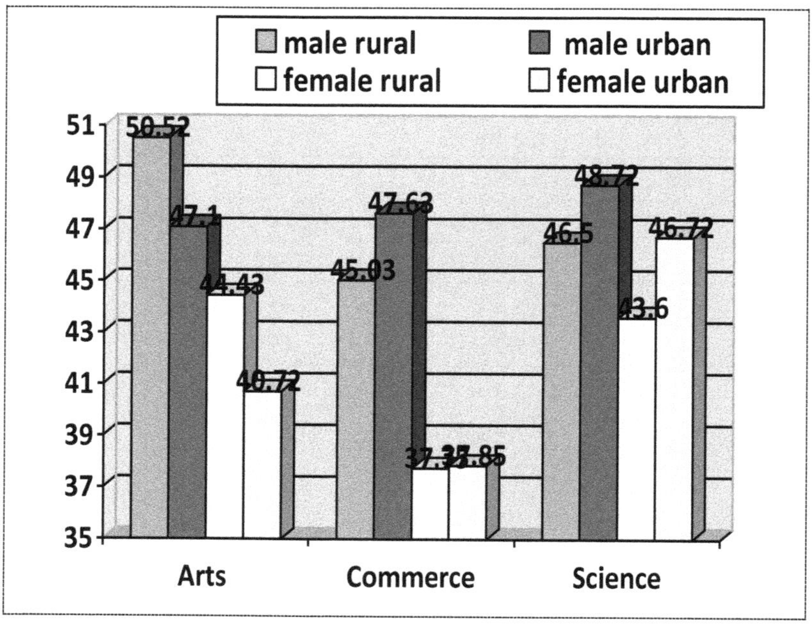

Figure No.07
Bar Chart of interaction between mean score of types of Faculty, sex and area variables on Internet Addiction

The table No.**4.3.15** indicated that the Interaction F for types of faculty, Sex and Area variables on Internet Addiction F value was **0.13**, which was not significance at **0.05** levels. Hence, the **Ho_8** was not rejected and it could be said that there was no significant mean difference between sex and area variables & their Internet Addiction score.

It could be seen from table No.**4.3.16** and **figure no.07** the all interaction means score and conclude that the urban male students are more Internet Addiction than other Area students. The highest mean score **33.04** was Urban male students. The present highest mean difference between $A_1B_1C_1$ vs. $A_2B_2C_1$ (Arts male rural and Commerce female rural) was 12.77, so it could be big difference. It was significant at 0.01 levels. The lowest mean difference between $A_2B_2C_1$ vs.$A_2B_2C_2$ (Commerce female rural vs. Commerce female urban) was 0.10 on Internet Addiction. It was not significant at 0.05 levels.

4.4.1 The Respondents socio personal variables and their 3x2x2 factorial design for Mental Health

Table No.4.4.1
The mean score for Independent variables on Mental Health

Variables	A1(Arts faculty)		A2(Commerce faculty)		A3(Science faculty)	
	B1 (male students)	B2 (female students)	B1 (male students)	B2 (female students)	B1 (male students)	B2 (female students)
C1 (Rural area)	∑X=5622 MX=93.7 N=60	∑X=5522 MX=92.03 N=60	∑X=5889 MX=98.15 N=60	∑X=5724 MX=95.4 N=60	∑X=5981 MX=99.68 N=60	∑X=5803 MX=96.72 N=60
C2 (Urban area)	∑X=5734 MX=95.57 N=60	∑X=5679 MX=94.65 N=60	∑X=5905 MX=98.42 N=60	∑X=5649 MX=94.15 N=60	∑X=5453 MX=90.88 N=60	∑X=5416 MX=90.27 N=60

The table no.**4.4.1** indicated the mean score for Independent variables on Mental Health. The highest mean score was 99.68 of rural male from Science faculty students and the lowest mean score was 90.27of urban female from Science faculty students. The mean score shows that Science male students from rural area were more Internet Addicted than other faculty students. The result also shows that Science female students from urban area were less Internet Addicted than other faculty students.

Table 4.4.2

F calculation for Mental Health (3x2x2 factorial designed)

Sources of variance	Sum of square	d.f.	Mean square	F	Significance level
Ass (Types of faculty)	936.99	2	468.50	4.39	0.05
Bss (Sex)	886.34	1	886.34	8.30	0.01
Css (Area)	614.24	1	614.24	5.75	0.05
ABss	158.82	2	79.41	0.74	N.S.
ACss	2885.09	2	1442.55	13.81	0.01
BCss	15.04	1	15.04	0.14	N.S.
ABCss	122.43	2	61.21	0.57	N.S.
Wss	75598.42	708	108.78	-	-
Tss	81278.27	719	-	-	-

Significance levels df_1 0.05 = 3.85, 0.01= 6.66
df_2 0.05 = 3.00, 0.01= 4.62

The table no.**4.4.2** point out that F value of Types of faculty variable was **4.39**, which was significance at **0.05** levels. The F value of sex variables was **8.30**, which was significance at **0.01** levels. The F value of Area variables was **5.75**, which was significance at **0.05** levels. The F value of Interaction to Types of faculty and Sex variables was **2.29**, which was not significance at **0.05** levels. The F value of Interaction to Types of faculty and Area variables was **2.54**, which was not significance at **0.05** levels.

The F value of Interaction to Sex and Area variables was **0.172**, which was not significance at **0.05** levels. The F value of Interaction to Types of faculty, Sex and Area variables was **0.13**.

Ho_8: There is no significance difference of Mental Health based on types of faculty variable.

Table No. 4.4.3
The mean and F value for Types of faculty variable on Mental Health

No.	Variables	N	Mean	F	Sig.
1	Arts faculty students (A_1)	240	94.01	**4.39**	**0.05**
2	Commerce faculty students(A_2)	240	96.53		
3	Science faculty students(A3)	240	94.37		

Significance levels df_2 = 0.05=3.00 / 0.01=4.63

Table No. 4.4.4
L.S.D. values for Types of faculty variable on Mental Health

Sr.No.	Pairs	Mean Diff.	Significance
1	A_1 vs. A_2	2.52	0.01
2	A_1 vs. A_3	0.36	N.S.
3	A_2 vs. A_3	2.16	0.05

Sig. levels for L.S.D. 0.05=1.85/ 0.01=2.43

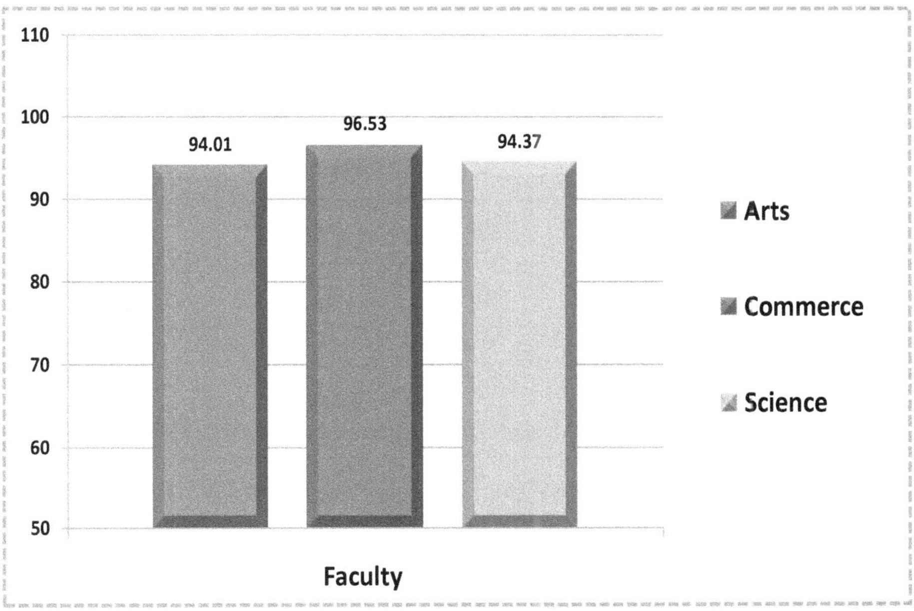

Figure No.08
Bar Chart of mean score of types of Faculty on Mental Health

The table no.**4.4.3** point out the mean score for the Arts faculty respondents were 94.01, the mean score of Commerce faculty respondents were 96.53 and the mean score of Science faculty respondents were 94.37. The F value for types of Faculty variable was 4.39 which were significant at 0.05 levels. Thus, Ho_8 was rejected at 0.05 levels. So it can say that there was significant difference between types of Faculty on Mental Health.

It could be seen from the table No.**4.4.4** and figure no.**08** L.S.D. values for types of faculty on Mental Health. The mean difference between Arts and Commerce faculty respondent was 2.52 which were significant at 0.01 levels. The mean difference between Arts and Science faculty respondent was 0.36, which was not significant at 0.05 levels. The mean difference between Commerce and Science respondents was 2.14, which was significant difference at 0.05 levels.

H_{0_9}: There is no significance difference of Mental Health based on Sex variables.

Table No 4.4.5

Mean score of Sex variables on Mental Health

Variables	N	Mean score	F	Sig.
B_1 (Male)	360	96.13	**8.30**	**0.01**
B_2 (Female)	360	93.87		

Significance levels df_2 =0.05=3.85 / 0.01=6.66

Table No. 4.4.6
L.S.D. values for Sex variable on Mental Health

No.	Variables(Sex)	N	Mean diff.	Significance
1	B_1 (Male)	360	2.33	0.01
2	B_2 (Female)	360		

Significance levels for L.S.D. =0.05=1.51/ 0.01=1.97

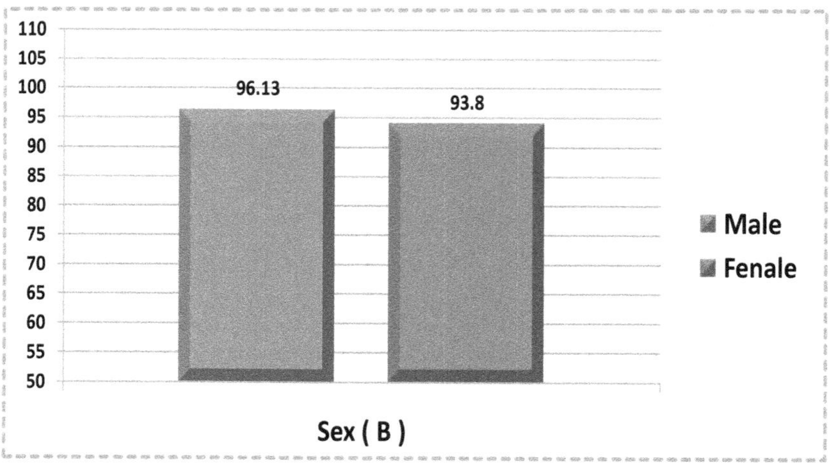

Figure No.09
Bar chart of mean score of sex variables on Mental Health

It is observed from the table No. **4.4.5** that the mean for male students was **96.13** and the mean for Female students was **93.80**. The F value for sex variables was **8.30,** which was significance at **0.01** levels. Hence, the **Ho_9** was rejected and it could be said that there was significant mean difference between types of sex & their Internet Addiction score. So it saw the result and said that the male students are more Internet addicted than female students. Hence it concluded that Internet Addiction was very affected factor for male students.

It could be seen from the table No. **4.4.6** and figure **No.08** the L.S.D. for Types of Sex variables on Mental Health that the mean different between Male and Female students on Mental Health was **2.33**, which was Significance at **0.01** levels. Thus it concluded that the Male students are more Mentally Healthy than Female students. Hence it concluded that Mental Health was very affected factor for Male students.

Ho_{10}: There is no significance difference of Mental Health on Area variables.

Table No.4.4.7

Mean score and F value of Area variables on Mental Health

Variables	N	Mean score	F	Sig.
C_1 (Rural)	360	95.90	**5.75**	**0.05**
C_2 (Urban)	360	94.03		

Significance levels df_2 =0.05=3.85/ 0.01=6.66

Table No. 4.4.8

L.S.D. values for Area variable on Mental Health

No.	Variables(Area)	N	Mean diff.	Sig.
1	Rural students (c_1)	360	**0.33**	**N.S.**
2	Urban students (c_2)	360		

Significance levels for L.S.D. =0.05=1.51/ 0.01=1.97

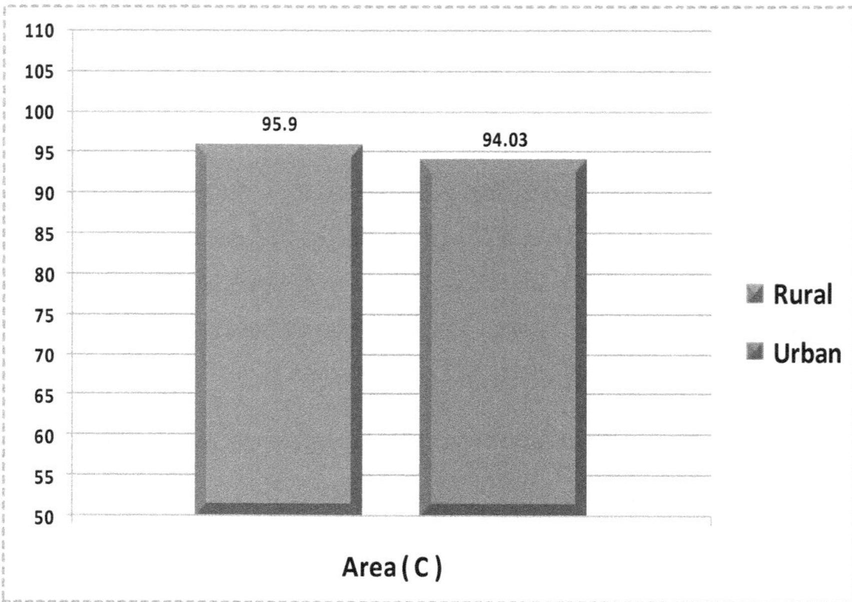

Figure No.10
Bar chart of mean score of Area variables on Mental Health

The table No. **4.4.7** indicated that the mean for rural students was **95.90** and the mean for urban students was **94.03**. The F value for **Area** variables was **5.75,** which was significance at **0.05** levels. Hence, the **Ho_{10}** was rejected and it could be said that there was significant mean difference between types of area & their Mental Health score.

It is observed from the table No. **4.4.8** and figure **No.10** the L.S.D. for types of Area variables on Mental Health that the mean different between Rural and Urban students on Mental Health was **0.33**, which was not Significant at **0.05** levels. Thus it concluded that the Rural students are more Mentally Healthy than Urban students. Hence it concluded that Mental Health was very affected factor for Male students.

Ho_{11}: There is no significance difference of Mental Health based on Interaction for types of faculty and Sex variables.

Table No 4.4.9
Interaction F for types of faculty and Sex variables on Mental Health

Variables	A_1 (Arts students)	A_2 (commerce students)	A_3 (Science students)	F	Sig.
B_1 (Male students)	94.63	98.28	95.28	0.74	N.S.
B_2 (Female students)	93.34	94.78	93.49		

Significance levels df2 =0.05=3.00 / 0.01=4.63

Table No 4.4.10
A L.S.D. Table for Interaction of Types of faculty and Sex variables on Mental Health

Sr.N0.	Pairs	Mean Diff.	Significance
1	A_1B_1 vs. A_1B_2	1.29	N.S.
2	A_1B_1 vs. A_2B_1	3.65	0.01
3	A_1B_1 vs. A_2B_2	0.15	N.S.
4	A_1B_1 vs. A_3B_1	0.65	N.S.
5	A_1B_1 vs. A_3B_2	1.14	N.S.
6	A_1B_2 vs. A_2B_1	4.94	0.01
7	A_1B_2 vs. A_2B_2	1.44	N.S.
8	A_1B_2 vs. A_3B_1	1.94	N.S.
9	A_1B_2 vs. A_3B_2	0.15	N.S.
10	A_2B_1 vs. A_2B_2	3.50	0.01
11	A_2B_1 vs. A_3B_1	3.00	0.05
12	A_2B_1 vs. A_3B_2	4.79	0.01
13	A_2B_2 vs. A_3B_1	0.50	N.S.
14	A_2B_2 vs. A_3B_2	1.29	N.S.
15	A_3B_1 vs. A_3B_2	1.79	N.S.

Sig. levels for L.S.D. 0.05=2.61/ 0.01=3.41

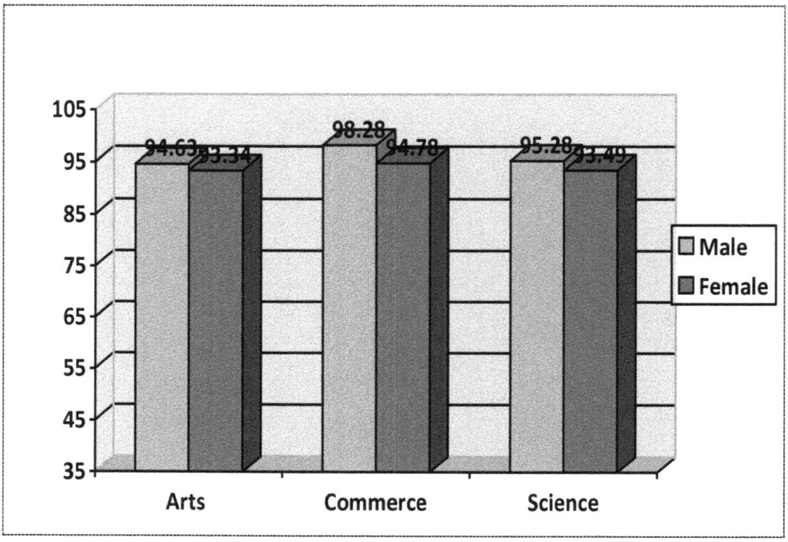

Figure No.11
Bar chart of mean score of Interaction of Types of faculty and Sex variables on Mental Health

It could be seen from the table No.**4.4.9** that the Interaction F for Types of faculty and Sex variables on Mental Health. The F value was **0.74**, which was not significance at **0.05** levels. Hence, the **Ho_{11}** was not rejected and it could be said that there was not significant mean difference between Types of faculty and sex variables & their Mental Health score.

Table no.**4.4.10** and figure **No.11** point out L.S.D. for interaction of types of faculty and sex variables on Mental Health. It could be seen from the result and said that most of the pairs are significance at 0.05 or 0.01 levels. It said that the highest mean score **98.28** was Commerce male students. The highest mean difference between A_1B_2 vs. A_2B_1 (Arts female students Vs. Commerce male students) was **4.94**, so it could be said that it was big difference. The lowest mean difference between A_1B_1 vs. A_2B_2 (Arts male students Vs. Commerce female students) was **0.15** on Mental Health. Hence, all the result concluded that either all variables (faculties and sex) are affected on Mental Health or Mental Health was affected them.

Ho_{12}: There is no significance difference of Mental Health based on Interaction for types of faculty and Area variables.

Table No 4.4.11

Interaction F for types of faculty and Area variables on Mental Health

Variables	A_1 (Arts faculty students)	A_2 (Commerce faculty students)	A_3 (Science faculty students)	F	Sig.
C_1 (Rural)	92.87	96.78	98.20	13.51	0.01
C_2 (Urban)	95.11	96.28	90.56		

Significance levels df2 =0.05=3.00 / 0.01=4.63

Table No 4.4.12

A L.S.D. Table for Interaction of Types of faculty and Area variables on Mental Health

Sr.N0.	Pairs	Mean Diff.	Significance
1	A_1C_1 vs. A_1C_2	2.24	N.S.
2	A_1C_1 vs. A_2C_1	3.91	0.01
3	A_1C_1 vs. A_2C_2	3.41	0.01
4	A_1C_1 vs.A_3C_1	5.33	0.01
5	A_1C_1 vs.A_3C_2	2.29	0.05
6	A_1C_2 vs. A_2C_1	1.67	N.S.
7	A_1C_2 vs. A_2C_2	1.17	N.S.
8	A_1C_2 vs. A_3C_1	3.09	0.05
9	A_1C_2 vs.A_3C_2	4.53	0.01
10	A_2C_1 vs.A_2C_2	0.50	N.S.
11	A_2C_1 vs.A_3C_1	1.42	N.S.
12	A_2C_1 vs.A_3C_2	8.20	0.01
13	A_2C_2 vs.A_3C_1	1.92	N.S.
14	A_2C_2 vs.A_3C_2	5.70	0.01
15	A_3C_1 vs.A_3C_2	7.62	0.01

Sig. levels for L.S.D. 0.05=2.61/ 0.01=3.41

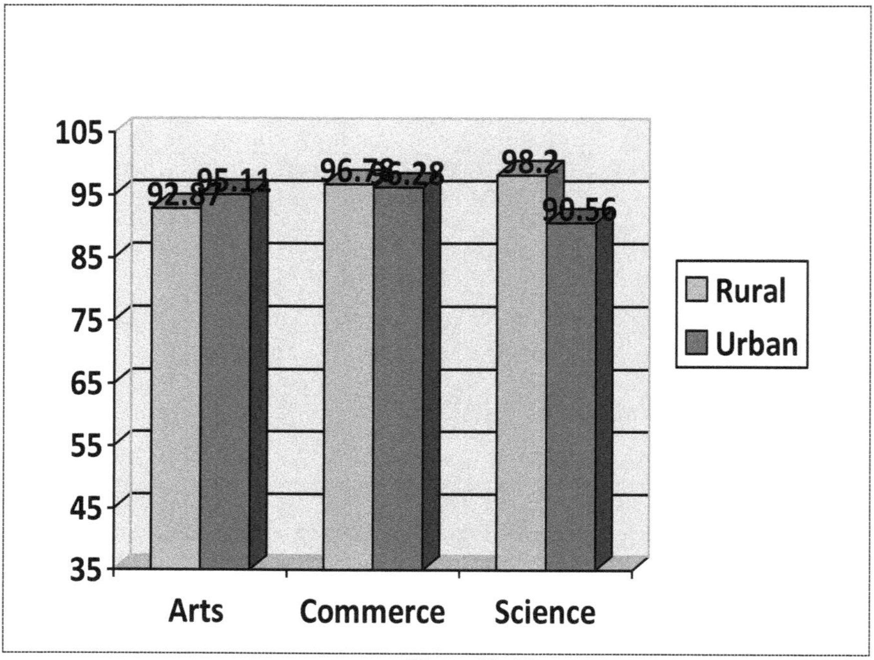

Figure No.12

Bar chart of interaction of Faculty and Area variables on Mental Health

It could be seen from the table No.**4.4.11** that the Interaction F for Types of faculty and Area variables on Mental Health. The F value was **13.51**, which was significance at **0.01** levels. Hence, the **Ho_{11}** was rejected and it could be said that there was significant mean difference between Types of faculty and area variables & their Mental Health score.

It is observed that the table no.**4.4.12** and figure **No.12** L.S.D. for interaction between the types of faculty and area variables on Mental Health. That it seen the result and said that the most of pairs significance at 0.05 or 0.01 levels. The highest mean difference between A_2C_1 vs.A_3C_2 (Commerce rural students Vs. Science urban students) was **8.20**, it was big difference. The lowest mean difference between A_2C_1 vs.A_2C_2 (Commerce rural students Vs. Commerce Urban students) was **0.50** on Mental Health.

Ho_{13}: There is no significance difference of Mental Health based on Interaction for Sex variables and Area variables

Table No 4.4.13
Interaction F for Sex variables and Area variables on Mental Health

Variables	B_1 (Male students)	B_2 (Female students)	F	Sig.
Rural students (C_1)	97.18	94.72	**0.14**	**N.S.**
Urban students (C_2)	94.96	94.69		

Significance levels df_2 =0.05=3.85 / 0.01=6.66

Table No 4.4.14
A L.S.D. Table for Interaction of Sex and Area variables on Mental Health

Sr.N0.	Pairs	Mean Diff.	Significance
1	B_1C_1 vs. B_1C_2	2.22	0.05
2	B_1C_1 vs. B_2C_1	2.46	0.05
3	B_1C_1 vs. B_2C_2	2.49	0.05
4	B_1C_2 vs. B_2C_1	0.24	N.S.
5	B_1C_2 vs. B_2C_2	0.27	N.S.
6	B_2C_1 vs. B_2C_2	0.03	N.S.

Sig. levels for L.S.D. 0.05=2.13/ 0.01=2.80

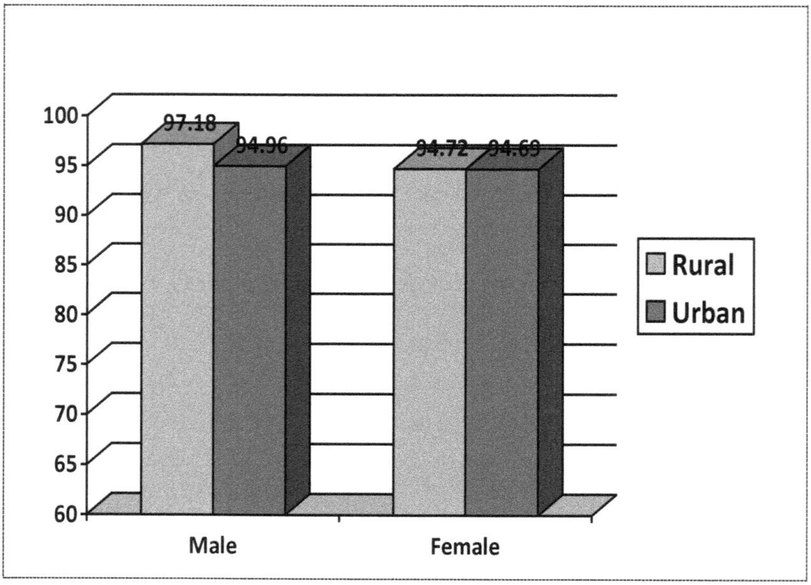

Figure No. 13
Bar chart of interaction between sex and area variables

Table No.**4.4.13** shows that the Interaction F for Sex variables and Area variables on Mental Health. F value was **0.14**, which was not significance at **0.05** levels. Hence, the **Ho$_{13}$** was not rejected at 0.05 levels and it could be said that there was no significant mean difference between Sex variables and Area variables & their Mental Health score.

It is observed from the table **4.4.14** and figure **No.13** L.S.D. for interaction between the Sex variables and Area variables on Mental Health, that it seen the result and said that most of pairs are significance at 0.05 levels. Highest mean difference between B_1C_1vs. B_2C_2 (male rural students Vs. female urban students) was 2.49, so it can said that it was big difference. The lowest mean difference score between B_2C_1 vs. B_2C_2 (female rural students vs. female urban students) was 0.03 on Mental Health.

Ho$_{14}$: There is no significance difference of Mental Health based on Interaction for types of faculty, Sex and Area variables.

Table No 4.4.15

Interaction F for types of Faculty, Sex and Area variables on Mental Health

	A_1(Arts students)		A_2(Commerce students)		A_3(Science students)		F	Sig.
	B_1 male students	B_2 female students	B_1 male students	B_2 female students	B_1 male students	B_2 female students		
C_1	93.7	92.03	98.15	95.4	99.68	96.72	0.53	N.S.
C_2	95.57	94.65	98.42	94.15	90.88	90.27		

Significance levels df_1 =0.05=3.00 / 0.01=4.63

Table No 4.4.16

A L.S.D. Table for Interaction of types of faculty, Sex and Area variables on Mental Health

Sr.N0.	Pairs	Mean Diff.	Significance
1	$A_1B_1C_1$ vs. $A_1B_1C_2$	1.87	N.S.
2	$A_1B_1C_1$ vs. $A_1B_2C_1$	1.67	N.S.
3	$A_1B_1C_1$ vs. $A_1B_2C_2$	0.95	N.S.
4	$A_1B_1C_1$ vs. $A_2B_1C_1$	4.45	0.05
5	$A_1B_1C_1$ vs. $A_2B_1C_2$	4.72	0.05
6	$A_1B_1C_1$ vs. $A_2B_2C_1$	1.72	N.S
7	$A_1B_1C_1$ vs. $A_2B_2C_2$	0.45	N.S
8	$A_1B_1C_1$ vs. $A_3B_1C_1$	5.98	0.01
9	$A_1B_1C_1$ vs. $A_3B_1C_2$	2.82	N.S
10	$A_1B_1C_1$ vs. $A_3B_2C_1$	3.02	N.S
11	$A_1B_1C_1$ vs. $A_3B_2C_2$	3.43	N.S.
12	$A_1B_1C_2$ vs. $A_1B_2C_1$	3.54	N.S.
13	$A_1B_1C_2$ vs. $A_1B_2C_2$	0.92	N.S.
14	$A_1B_1C_2$ vs. $A_2B_1C_1$	2.58	N.S.
15	$A_1B_1C_2$ vs. $A_2B_1C_2$	2.85	N.S.
16	$A_1B_1C_2$ vs. $A_2B_2C_1$	0.17	N.S.
17	$A_1B_1C_2$ vs. $A_2B_2C_2$	1.42	N.S.

18	$A_1B_1C_2$ vs. $A_3B_1C_1$	4.11	0.05
19	$A_1B_1C_2$ vs. $A_3B_1C_2$	4.69	0.05
20	$A_1B_1C_2$ vs. $A_3B_2C_1$	1.15	N.S.
21	$A_1B_1C_2$ vs. $A_3B_2C_2$	5.3	0.01
22	$A_1B_2C_1$ vs. $A_1B_2C_2$	2.62	N.S.
23	$A_1B_2C_1$ vs. $A_2B_1C_1$	6.12	0.01
24	$A_1B_2C_1$ vs. $A_2B_1C_2$	6.39	0.01
25	$A_1B_2C_1$ vs. $A_2B_2C_1$	3.37	N.S.
26	$A_1B_2C_1$ vs. $A_2B_2C_2$	2.12	N.S.
27	$A_1B_2C_1$ vs. $A_3B_1C_1$	7.65	0.01
28	$A_1B_2C_1$ vs. $A_3B_1C_2$	1.15	N.S.
29	$A_1B_2C_1$ vs. $A_3B_2C_1$	4.69	0.05
30	$A_1B_2C_1$ vs. $A_3B_2C_2$	1.76	N.S.
31	$A_1B_2C_2$ vs. $A_2B_1C_1$	3.5	N.S.
32	$A_1B_2C_2$ vs. $A_2B_1C_2$	3.77	0.05
33	$A_1B_2C_2$ vs. $A_2B_2C_1$	0.75	N.S.
34	$A_1B_2C_2$ vs. $A_2B_2C_2$	0.50	N.S.
35	$A_1B_2C_2$ vs. $A_3B_1C_1$	5.03	0.01
36	$A_1B_2C_2$ vs. $A_3B_1C_2$	3.71	0.05
37	$A_1B_2C_2$ vs. $A_3B_2C_1$	2.07	N.S.
38	$A_1B_2C_2$ vs. $A_3B_2C_2$	4.38	0.05
39	$A_2B_1C_1$ vs. $A_2B_1C_2$	0.27	N.S.
40	$A_2B_1C_1$ vs. $A_2B_2C_1$	2.75	N.S.
41	$A_2B_1C_1$ vs. $A_2B_2C_2$	4.00	0.01
42	$A_2B_1C_1$ vs. $A_3B_1C_1$	1.53	N.S.
43	$A_2B_1C_1$ vs. $A_3B_1C_2$	7.27	0.01
44	$A_2B_1C_1$ vs. $A_3B_2C_1$	1.43	N.S.
45	$A_2B_1C_1$ vs. $A_3B_2C_2$	7.88	0.01
46	$A_2B_1C_2$ vs. $A_2B_2C_1$	3.02	N.S.
47	$A_2B_1C_2$ vs. $A_2B_2C_2$	4.27	0.05
48	$A_2B_1C_2$ vs. $A_3B_1C_1$	1.26	N.S.
49	$A_2B_1C_2$ vs. $A_3B_1C_2$	7.54	0.01
50	$A_2B_1C_2$ vs. $A_3B_2C_1$	1.7	N.S.

51	$A_2B_1C_2$ vs. $A_3B_2C_2$	8.15	0.01
52	$A_2B_2C_1$ vs. $A_2B_2C_2$	1.25	N.S.
53	$A_2B_2C_1$ vs. $A_3B_1C_1$	4.28	0.05
54	$A_2B_2C_1$ vs. $A_3B_1C_2$	4.52	0.05
55	$A_2B_2C_1$ vs. $A_3B_2C_1$	1.32	N.S.
56	$A_2B_2C_1$ vs. $A_3B_2C_2$	5.13	0.01
57	$A_2B_2C_2$ vs. $A_3B_1C_1$	5.53	0.01
58	$A_2B_2C_2$ vs. $A_3B_1C_2$	3.27	N.S.
59	$A_2B_2C_2$ vs. $A_3B_2C_1$	2.57	N.S.
60	$A_2B_2C_2$ vs. $A_3B_2C_2$	3.88	0.05
61	$A_3B_1C_1$ vs. $A_3B_1C_2$	8.8	0.01
62	$A_3B_1C_1$ vs. $A_3B_2C_1$	2.96	N.S.
63	$A_3B_1C_1$ vs. $A_3B_2C_2$	9.41	0.01
64	$A_3B_1C_2$ vs. $A_3B_2C_1$	5.84	0.01
65	$A_3B_1C_2$vs. $A_3B_2C_2$	0.61	N.S.
66	$A_3B_2.C_1$ vs. $A_3B_2C_2$	6.45	0.01

Sig. levels for L.S.D. 0.05=3.70 / 0.01=4.86

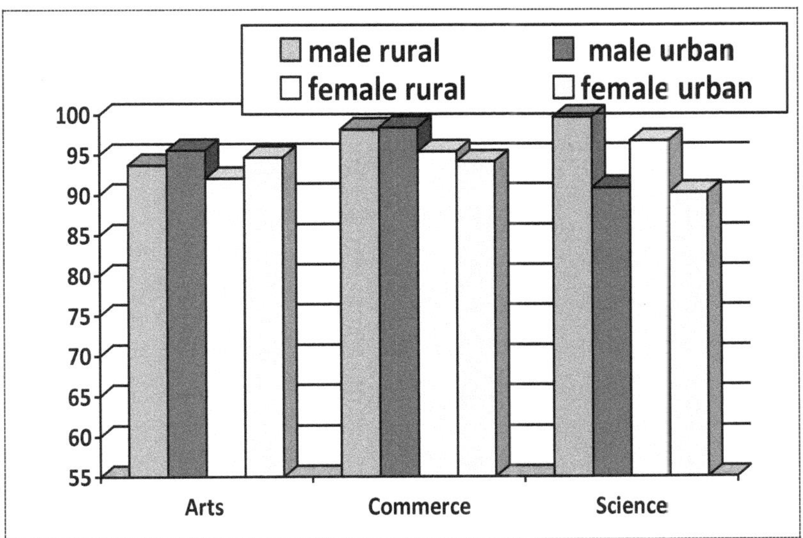

Figure No.14
The bar chart for interaction between the types of faculty, sex and area variables on Mental Health

It could be seen from the table No.**4.4.15** that the Interaction F for Sex and Area variables on Mental Health. F value was **0.53,** which was not significance at **0.05** levels. Hence, the **Ho_{14}** was not rejected and it could be said that there was no significant mean difference between sex and area variables & their Mental Health score. It is observed that the all interaction means score and conclude that the Science Rural male students got more score in Mental Health than other students. The highest mean score **99.68** was Science Rural male students.

Table No.4.4.16 and figure No.14 indicated the LSD values of interaction three independent variables on Mental Health. Highest mean difference between $A_2B_2C_2$ vs. $A_3B_2C_2$ was 8.8, it was a big difference. The lowest mean difference between $A_1B_1C_2$ vs. $A_2B_1C_2$ was 0.17 on Mental Health.

4.5.1 The Respondents socio personal variables and their 3x2x2 factorial design for Perception of reality a part of mental health

Table No.4.5.1
The mean score for Independent variables on Perception of reality a part of mental health

Variables	A1(Arts faculty)		A2(Commerce faculty)		A3(Science faculty)	
	B1 male students	B2 female students	B1 male students	B2 female students	B1 male students	B2 female students
C1 (Rural area)	∑X=1110 MX=18.5 N=60	∑X=1072 MX=17.87 N=60	∑X=1157 MX=19.2 8 N=60	∑X=1147 MX=19.12 N=60	∑X=1185 MX=19.75 N=60	∑X=1145 MX=19.08 N=60
C2 (Urban area)	∑X=1136 MX=18.93 N=60	∑X=1109 MX=18.48 N=60	∑X=1189 MX=19.82 N=60	∑X=1151 MX=19.18 N=60	∑X=1111 MX=18.52 N=60	∑X=1082 MX=18.03 N=60

It could be seen from the table No.**4.5.1** the mean score for Independent variables on Mental Health. The highest mean score was 19.82 of urban male from Commerce faculty students and the lowest mean score was 17.87 of rural female from Arts faculty students.

Table 4.5.2

F calculation for Perception of reality a part of mental health (3x2x2 factorial designed)

Sources of variance	Sum of square	d.f.	Mean square	F	Significance level
Ass (Types of faculty)	98.72	2	49.36	8.08	0.01
Bss (Sex)	45.29	1	45.29	7.41	0.01
Css (Area)	1.69	1	01.69	0.28	N.S.
ABss	0.98	2	00.49	0.08	N.S.
ACss	96.48	2	48.24	7.90	0.01
BCss	0.04	1	00.04	0.01	N.S.
ABCss	5.86	2	02.93	0.48	N.S.
Wss	4325.89	708	06.11	-	-
Tss	4577.73	719	-	-	-

Significance levels df_1 0.05 = 3.85, 0.01= 6.66
df_2 0.05 = 3.00, 0.01= 4.62

It is observed from the table no.**4.5.2** that F value of types of faculty variable was **8.08**, which was significance at **0.01** levels. The F value of sex variables was 7.41, which was significance at **0.01** levels. The F value of Area variables was **0.28**, which was not significance at **0.05** levels. The F value of Interaction to types of faculty and Sex variables was **0.08**, which was not significance at **0.05** levels. The F value of Interaction to types of faculty and Area variables was **7.90**, which was significance at **0.01** levels.

The F value of Interaction to Sex and Area variables was **0.01**, which was not significance at **0.05** levels. The F value of Interaction to types of faculty, Sex and Area variables was **0.48**.

Ho_{15}: There is no significance difference of Perception of reality a part of Mental Health based on types of faculty variable.

Table No. 4.5.3
The mean and F value for Types of faculty variable on Perception of reality types Mental Health

No.	Variables	N	Mean	F	Significance
1	Arts faculty students (A_1)	240	18.45	**8.08**	**0.01**
2	Commerce faculty students(A_2)	240	19.35		
3	Science faculty students(A3)	240	18.84		

Significance levels df_2 = 0.05=3.00 / 0.01=4.63

Table No. 4.5.4
L.S.D. value for Types of faculty variable on Perception of reality a part of Mental Health

Sr.No.	Pairs	Mean Diff.	Significance
1	A_1 vs. A_2	0.90	0.01
2	A_1 vs. A_3	0.39	N.S.
3	A_2 vs. A_3	0.51	0.05

Sig. levels for L.S.D. 0.05=0.44/0.01=0.58

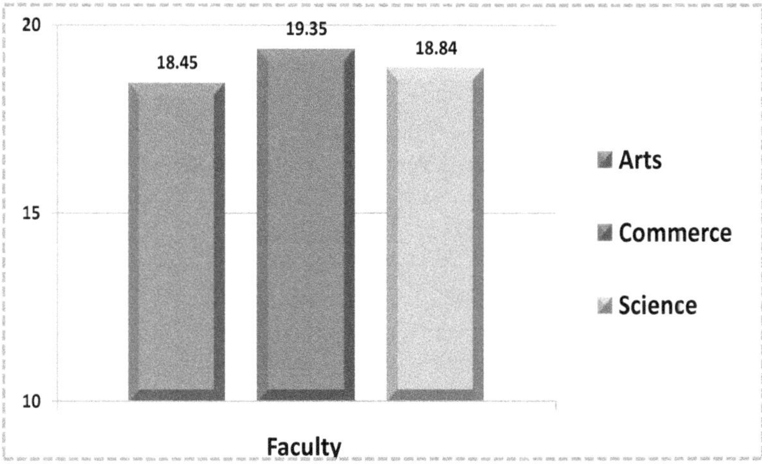

Figure No.15
Bar Chart of mean score of types of Faculty on Perception of reality a part of Mental Health

The table no.**4.5.3** shows the mean score for the Arts faculty respondents were 18.45, the mean score of Commerce faculty respondents were 19.35 and the mean score of Science faculty respondents were 18.84. The F value for types of Faculty variable was 8.08 which was significant at 0.01 levels. Thus, our Ho_{15} was rejected at 0.01 levels. So it can say that there was significant difference between types of Faculty on Perception of reality types Mental Health.

It is observed from the table No.**4.5.4** and figure no.**15** L.S.D. values for types of faculty on Perception of reality types Mental Health. The mean difference between Arts and Commerce faculty respondent was 0.9 which were significant at 0.01 levels. The mean difference between Arts and Science faculty respondent was 0.39, which was not significant at 0.05 levels. The mean difference between Commerce and Science respondents was 0.51, which was significant difference at 0.05 levels.

Ho_{16}: There is no significance difference of Perception of reality a part of Mental Health based on Sex variables.

Table No 4.5.5
Mean score of Sex variables on Perception of reality a part of Mental Health

Variables	N	Mean score	F	Sig.
B_1 (Male)	360	19.14	**7.41**	**0.01**
B_2 (Female)	360	18.62		

Significance levels df_2 =0.05=3.85 / 0.01=6.66

Table No. 4.5.6
L.S.D. value for Sex variable on Perception of reality a part of Mental Health

No.	Variables(Sex)	N	Mean diff.	Significance
1	B_1 (Male)	360	0.52	0.01
2	B_2 (Female)	360		

Significance levels for L.S.D. =0.05=0.35 / 0.01=0.46

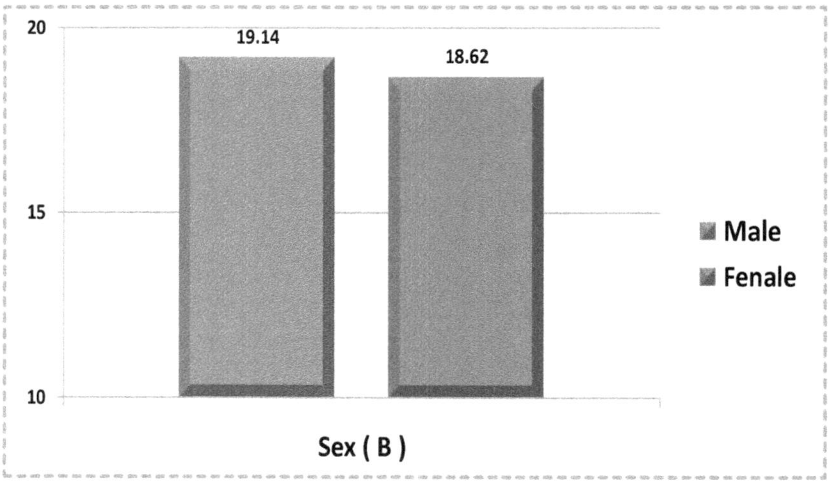

Figure No.16
Bar chart of mean score of sex variables on Perception of reality a part of Mental Health

It could be seen from the table No. **4.5.5** that the mean for male students was **19.14** and the mean for Female students was **18.62**. The F value for sex variables was **7.41,** which was significance at **0.01** levels. Hence, the **Ho_{16}** was rejected and it could be said that there was significant mean difference between types of sex & their Perception of reality types Mental Health score. So it saw the result and said that the male students are more Perception of reality types Mental Health than female students. Hence it concluded that Perception of reality types Mental Health was very affected factor for male students.

The table No. **4.5.6** and figure **No.16** point out the L.S.D. for Types of Sex variables on Perception of reality types Mental Health that the mean different between Male and Female students on Perception of reality types Mental Health was **0.52**, which was Significance at **0.01** levels. Thus it concluded that the Male students are more Perception of reality types Mentally Healthy than Female students. Hence it concluded that Mental Health was very affected factor for Male students.

Ho_{17}: There is no significance difference of Perception of reality a part of Mental Health on Area variables.

Table No 4.5.7
Mean score and F value of Area variables on Perception of reality a part of Mental Health

Variables	N	Mean score	F	Sig.
C_1 (Rural)	360	18.93	**0.27**	**N.S.**
C_2 (Urban)	360	18.83		

Significance levels df_2 =0.05=3.85/ 0.01=6.66

Table No. 4.5.8
L.S.D. value for Area variable on Perception of reality a part of Mental Health

No.	Variables(Area)	N	Mean diff.	Significance
1	Rural students (c_1)	360	**0.10**	**N.S.**
2	Urban students (c_2)	360		

Significance levels for L.S.D. =0.05=0.55

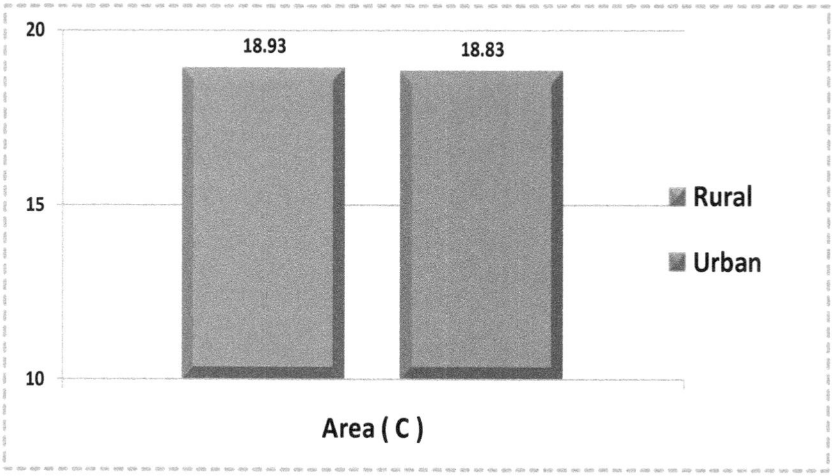

Figure No.17
Bar chart of mean score of Area variables on Perception of reality a part of Mental Health

The table No. **4.5.7** point out that the mean for rural students was **18.93** and the mean for urban students was **18.83**. The F value for Area variables was **0.27,** which was not significance at **0.05** levels. Hence, the **Ho_{17}** was not rejected and it could be said that there was no significant mean difference between types of area & their Perception of reality types Mental Health score.

It could be seen from the table No. 4.5.8 and figure No.17 the L.S.D. for types of Area variables on Perception of reality types Mental Health that the mean different between Rural and Urban students on Mental Health was **0.10**, which was not Significant at **0.05** levels. Thus it concluded that the Rural students are more Perception of reality types Mentally Healthy than Urban students. Hence it concluded that Perception of reality types Mental Health was very affected factor for Male students.

Ho_{18}: There is no significance difference of Perception of reality a part of Mental Health based on Interaction for types of faculty and Sex variables.

Table No 4.5.9

Interaction F for types of faculty and Sex variables on Perception of reality a part of Mental Health

Variables	A_1 Arts students	A_2 commerce students	A_3 Science students	F	Sig.
B_1 (Male students)	**18.72**	**19.55**	**19.13**	**0.08**	**N.S.**
B_2 (Female students)	**18.18**	**19.15**	**18.56**		

Significance levels df2 =0.05=3.00 / 0.01=4.63

Table No 4.5.10

A L.S.D. Table for Interaction of Types of faculty and Sex variables on Perception of reality a part of Mental Health

Sr.N0.	Pairs	Mean Diff.	Significance
1	A_1B_1 vs. A_1B_2	0.54	N.S.
2	A_1B_1 vs. A_2B_1	0.83	0.01
3	A_1B_1 vs. A_2B_2	0.43	N.S.
4	A_1B_1 vs. A_3B_1	0.41	N.S.
5	A_1B_1 vs. A_3B_2	0.16	N.S.
6	A_1B_2 vs. A_2B_1	1.37	0.01
7	A_1B_2 vs. A_2B_2	0.97	0.01
8	A_1B_2 vs. A_3B_1	0.95	0.01
9	A_1B_2 vs. A_3B_2	0.38	N.S.
10	A_2B_1 vs. A_2B_2	0.40	N.S.
11	A_2B_1 vs. A_3B_1	0.42	N.S.
12	A_2B_1 vs. A_3B_2	0.99	0.01
13	A_2B_2 vs. A_3B_1	0.02	N.S.
14	A_2B_2 vs. A_3B_2	0.59	N.S.
15	A_3B_1 vs. A_3B_2	0.57	N.S.

Sig. levels for L.S.D. 0.05=0.63 / 0.01=0.83

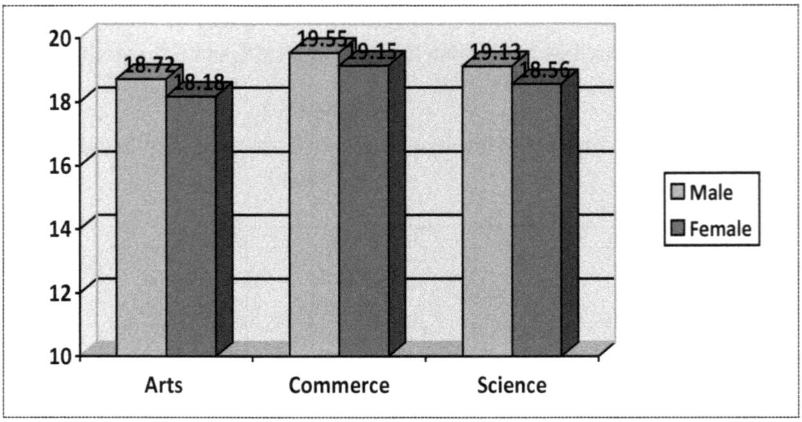

Figure No.18
Bar chart of mean score of Interaction of Types of faculty and Sex variables on Perception of reality a part of Mental Health

It is observed from the table No.**4.43** that the Interaction F for Types of faculty and Sex variables on Perception of reality types Mental Health. The F value was **0.08**, which was not significance at **0.05** levels. Hence, the $\mathbf{Ho_{18}}$ was not rejected and it could be said that there was not significant mean difference between Types of faculty and sex variables & their Perception of reality types Mental Health score.

The table no.**4.5.10** and figure **No.18** indicated L.S.D. for interaction of types of faculty and sex variables on Perception of reality types Mental Health. The result said that most of the pairs are significance at 0.05 or 0.01 levels. It also said that the highest mean score **19.55** was Commerce male students. The highest mean difference between A_1B_2 vs. A_2B_1 (Arts female students Vs. Commerce male students) was **1.37**, so it was big difference. The lowest mean difference between A_2B_2 vs. A_3B_1(Arts male students Vs. Commerce female students) was **0.02** on Perception of reality types Mental Health. Hence, we see all the result and concluded that either all variables (faculties and sex) are affected on Perception of reality types Mental Health or Perception of reality types Mental Health was affected them.

Ho_{19}: There is no significance difference of Perception of reality a part of Mental Health based on Interaction for types of faculty and Area variables.

Table No 4.5.11
Interaction F for types of faculty and Area variables on Perception of reality a part of Mental Health

Variables	A_1 (Arts students)	A_2 (Commerce students)	A_3 (Science students)	F	Sig.
C_1 (Rural)	**18.18**	**19.20**	**19.42**	**7.90**	**0.01**
C_2 (Urban)	**18.71**	**19.50**	**18.28**		

Significance levels df2 =0.05=3.00 / 0.01=4.63

Table No 4.5.12
A L.S.D. Table for Interaction of Types of faculty and Area variables on Perception of reality types Mental Health

Sr.N0.	Pairs	Mean Diff.	Significance
1	A_1C_1 vs. A_1C_2	0.53	N.S.
2	A_1C_1 vs. A_2C_1	1.02	0.01
3	A_1C_1 vs. A_2C_2	1.32	0.01
4	A_1C_1 vs.A_3C_1	1.24	0.01
5	A_1C_1 vs.A_3C_2	0.10	N.S.
6	A_1C_2 vs. A_2C_1	0.49	N.S.
7	A_1C_2 vs. A_2C_2	0.79	0.05
8	A_1C_2 vs. A_3C_1	0.71	0.05
9	A_1C_2 vs.A_3C_2	0.43	N.S.
10	A_2C_1 vs.A_2C_2	0.30	N.S.
11	A_2C_1 vs.A_3C_1	0.22	N.S.
12	A_2C_1 vs.A_3C_2	0.92	0.01
13	A_2C_2 vs.A_3C_1	0.08	N.S.
14	A_2C_2 vs.A_3C_2	1.22	0.01
15	A_3C_1 vs.A_3C_2	1.14	0.01

Sig. levels for L.S.D. 0.05=0.63/ 0.01=0.83

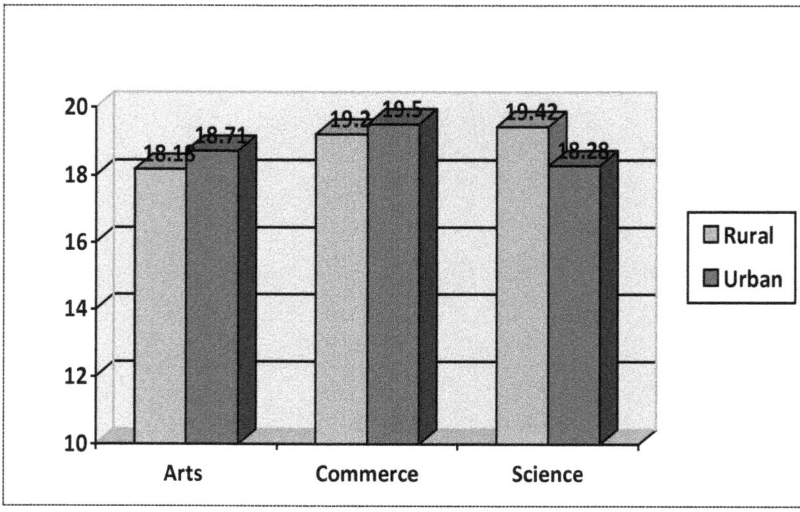

Figure No.19
Bar chart of interaction of Faculty and Area variables on Perception of reality a part of Mental Health

It could be seen from the table No.**4.5.11** that the Interaction F for types of faculty and Area variables on Perception of reality a part of mental health. The F value was **7.90**, which was significance at **0.01** levels. Hence, the **Ho_{19}** was rejected and it could be said that there was significant mean difference between types of faculty and area variables & their Perception of reality a part of mental health score.

It is observed from the no.**4.5.12** and figure No.19 L.S.D. for interaction between the types of faculty and area variables on Perception of reality a part of mental health. That the result points out that the most of pairs significance at 0.05 or 0.01 levels. It also said the highest mean difference between A_1C_1 vs. A_2C_2 (Arts rural students Vs. Commerce urban students) was **1.32**, so we can say that it was big difference. The lowest mean difference between A_2C_2vs.A_3C_1 (Commerce urban students Vs. Science rural students) was **0.08** on Perception of reality a part of mental health.

Ho_{20}: There is no significance difference of Perception of reality a part of mental health based on Interaction for Sex variables and Area variables.

Table No 4.5.13

Interaction F for Sex variables and Area variables on Perception of reality a part of mental health

Variables	B_1 (Male students)	B_2 (Female students)	F	Sig.
Rural students (C_1)	19.18	18.69	**0.01**	**N.S.**
Urban students (C_2)	19.09	18.57		

Significance levels df_2 =0.05=3.85/ 0.01=6.66

Table No 4.5.14

A L.S.D. Table for Interaction of Sex and Area variables on Perception of reality a part of mental health

Sr.N0.	Pairs	Mean Diff.	Significance
1	B_1C_1 vs. B_1C_2	0.09	N.S.
2	B_1C_1 vs. B_2C_1	0.49	N.S.
3	B_1C_1 vs. B_2C_2	0.61	0.05
4	B_1C_2 vs.B_2C_1	0.40	N.S.
5	B_1C_2 vs. B_2C_2	0.52	0.05
6	B_2C_1 vs. B_2C_2	0.12	N.S.

Sig. levels for L.S.D. 0.05=0.51 / 0.01=0.67

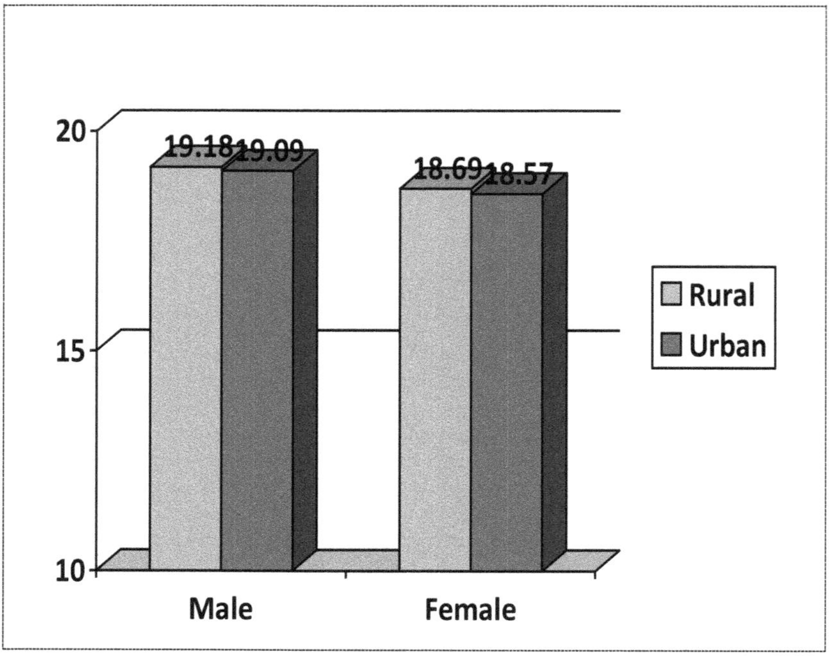

Figure No. 20
Bar chart of interaction of Sex and Area variables on Perception of reality a part of Mental Health

It is observed from the table No.**4.5.13** that the Interaction F for Sex variables and Area variables on Perception of reality a part of Mental Health. F value was **0.01**, which was not significance at **0.05** levels. Hence, the $\mathbf{Ho_{20}}$ was not rejected at 0.05 levels and it could be said that there was no significant mean difference between Sex variables and Area variables & their Perception of reality a part of Mental Health score.

The table **4.5.14** and figure **No.20** shows L.S.D. for interaction between the Sex variables and Area variables on Perception of reality types Mental Health, that it seen the result and said that most of pairs are significance at 0.05 levels. It also said highest mean difference between B_1C_1vs. B_2C_2 (male rural students vs. female urban students) was 0.61, so it said that it was big difference. The lowest mean difference score between B_2C_1 vs. B_2C_2 (female rural students vs. female urban students) was 0.12on Perception of reality a part of Mental Health.

Ho_{21}: There is no significance difference of Perception of reality a part of Mental Health based on Interaction for types of faculty, Sex and Area variables

Table No 4.5.15

Interaction F for types of Faculty, Sex and Area variables on Perception of reality a part of Mental Health

variables	A_1(Arts students)		A_2(Commerce students)		A_3(Science students)		F	Signi.
	B_1 male students	B_2 female students	B_1 male students	B_2 female students	B_1 male students	B_2 female students		
C_1	18.5	17.87	19.28	19.12	19.75	19.08	0.48	N.S.
C_2	18.93	18.48	19.82	19.18	18.52	18.03		

Significance levels df_1 =0.05=3.00 / 0.01=4.63

Table No 4.5.16

A L.S.D. Table for Interaction of types of faculty, Sex and Area variables on Perception of reality a part of Mental Health

Sr.No.	Pairs	Mean Diff.	Significance
1	$A_1B_1C_1$ vs. $A_1B_1C_2$	0.43	N.S.
2	$A_1B_1C_1$ vs. $A_1B_2C_1$	0.63	N.S.
3	$A_1B_1C_1$ vs. $A_1B_2C_2$	0.02	N.S.
4	$A_1B_1C_1$ vs. $A_2B_1C_1$	0.78	N.S.
5	$A_1B_1C_1$ vs. $A_2B_1C_2$	1.32	0.01
6	$A_1B_1C_1$ vs. $A_2B_2C_1$	0.62	N.S.
7	$A_1B_1C_1$ vs. $A_2B_2C_2$	0.68	N.S.
8	$A_1B_1C_1$ vs. $A_3B_1C_1$	1.25	0.01
9	$A_1B_1C_1$ vs. $A_3B_1C_2$	0.02	N.S.
10	$A_1B_1C_1$ vs. $A_3B_2C_1$	0.58	N.S.
11	$A_1B_1C_1$ vs. $A_3B_2C_2$	0.47	N.S.
12	$A_1B_1C_2$ vs. $A_1B_2C_1$	1.06	0.05
13	$A_1B_1C_2$ vs. $A_1B_2C_2$	0.45	N.S.
14	$A_1B_1C_2$ vs. $A_2B_1C_1$	0.35	N.S.
15	$A_1B_1C_2$ vs. $A_2B_1C_2$	0.89	0.05

16	$A_1B_1C_2$ vs. $A_2B_2C_1$	0.19	N.S.
17	$A_1B_1C_2$ vs. $A_2B_2C_2$	0.25	N.S.
18	$A_1B_1C_2$ vs. $A_3B_1C_1$	0.82	N.S.
19	$A_1B_1C_2$ vs. $A_3B_1C_2$	0.59	N.S.
20	$A_1B_1C_2$ vs. $A_3B_2C_1$	0.15	N.S.
21	$A_1B_1C_2$ vs. $A_3B_2C_2$	0.90	0.05
22	$A_1B_2C_1$ vs. $A_1B_2C_2$	0.61	N.S.
23	$A_1B_2C_1$ vs. $A_2B_1C_1$	1.41	0.01
24	$A_1B_2C_1$ vs. $A_2B_1C_2$	1.95	0.01
25	$A_1B_2C_1$ vs. $A_2B_2C_1$	1.25	0.01
26	$A_1B_2C_1$ vs. $A_2B_2C_2$	1.31	0.01
27	$A_1B_2C_1$ vs. $A_3B_1C_1$	1.88	0.01
28	$A_1B_2C_1$ vs. $A_3B_1C_2$	0.65	N.S.
29	$A_1B_2C_1$ vs. $A_3B_2C_1$	1.21	0.01
30	$A_1B_2C_1$ vs. $A_3B_2C_2$	0.16	N.S.
31	$A_1B_2C_2$ vs. $A_2B_1C_1$	0.80	N.S.
32	$A_1B_2C_2$ vs. $A_2B_1C_2$	1.34	0.01
33	$A_1B_2C_2$ vs. $A_2B_2C_1$	0.64	N.S.
34	$A_1B_2C_2$ vs. $A_2B_2C_2$	0.70	N.S.
35	$A_1B_2C_2$ vs. $A_3B_1C_1$	1.27	0.01
36	$A_1B_2C_2$ vs. $A_3B_1C_2$	0.04	N.S.
37	$A_1B_2C_2$ vs. $A_3B_2C_1$	0.60	N.S.
38	$A_1B_2C_2$ vs. $A_3B_2C_2$	0.45	N.S.
39	$A_2B_1C_1$ vs. $A_2B_1C_2$	0.54	N.S.
40	$A_2B_1C_1$ vs. $A_2B_2C_1$	0.16	N.S.
41	$A_2B_1C_1$ vs. $A_2B_2C_2$	0.10	N.S.
42	$A_2B_1C_1$ vs. $A_3B_1C_1$	0.47	N.S.
43	$A_2B_1C_1$ vs. $A_3B_1C_2$	0.76	N.S.
44	$A_2B_1C_1$ vs. $A_3B_2C_1$	0.20	N.S.
45	$A_2B_1C_1$ vs. $A_3B_2C_2$	1.25	0.01
46	$A_2B_1C_2$ vs. $A_2B_2C_1$	0.70	N.S.
47	$A_2B_1C_2$ vs. $A_2B_2C_2$	0.64	N.S.
48	$A_2B_1C_2$ vs. $A_3B_1C_1$	0.07	N.S.

49	$A_2B_1C_2$ vs. $A_3B_1C_2$	1.30	0.01
50	$A_2B_1C_2$ vs. $A_3B_2C_1$	0.74	N.S.
51	$A_2B_1C_2$ vs. $A_3B_2C_2$	1.79	0.01
52	$A_2B_2C_1$ vs. $A_2B_2C_2$	0.06	N.S.
53	$A_2B_2C_1$ vs. $A_3B_1C_1$	0.63	N.S.
54	$A_2B_2C_1$ vs. $A_3B_1C_2$	0.60	N.S.
55	$A_2B_2C_1$ vs. $A_3B_2C_1$	0.04	N.S.
56	$A_2B_2C_1$ vs. $A_3B_2C_2$	1.09	0.05
57	$A_2B_2C_2$ vs. $A_3B_1C_1$	0.57	N.S.
58	$A_2B_2C_2$ vs. $A_3B_1C_2$	0.66	N.S.
59	$A_2B_2C_2$ vs. $A_3B_2C_1$	0.10	N.S.
60	$A_2B_2C_2$ vs. $A_3B_2C_2$	1.15	0.01
61	$A_3B_1C_1$ vs. $A_3B_1C_2$	1.23	0.01
62	$A_3B_1C_1$ vs. $A_3B_2C_1$	0.67	N.S.
63	$A_3B_1C_1$ vs. $A_3B_2C_2$	1.72	0.01
64	$A_3B_1C_2$ vs. $A_3B_2C_1$	0.56	N.S.
65	$A_3B_1C_2$vs. $A_3B_2C_2$	0.49	N.S.
66	$A_3B_2.C_1$ vs. $A_3B_2C_2$	1.05	0.05

Sig.levels for L.S.D. 0.05=0.88 / 0.01=1.16

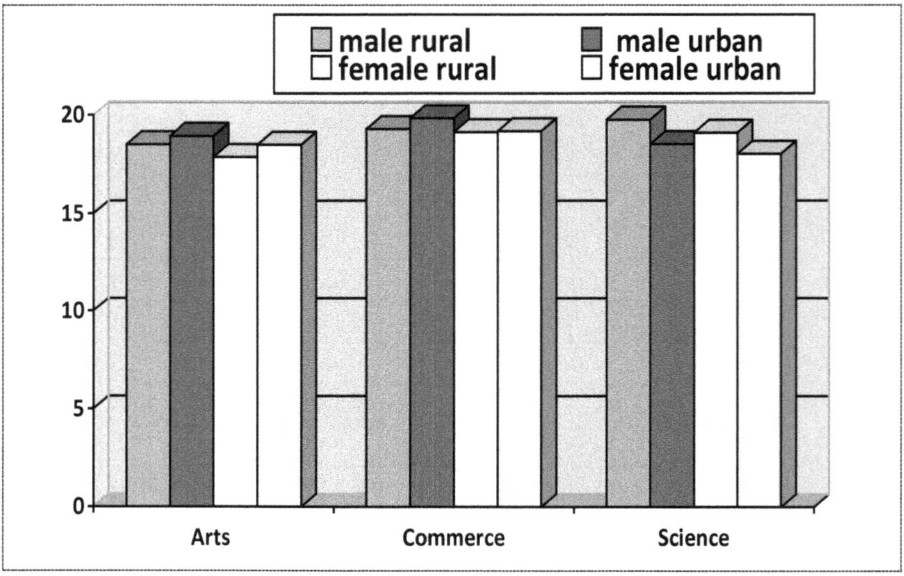

Figure No.21
The bar chart of interaction between the types of faculty, sex and area variables on Perception of reality a part of mental health

It could be seen from the table No.**4.5.15** that the Interaction F for Sex and Area variables on Perception of reality a part of Mental Health. F value was **0.48,** which was not significance at **0.05** levels. Hence, the **Ho**$_{14}$ was not rejected and it could be said that there was no significant mean difference between sex and area variables & their Perception of reality a part of Mental Health score.

It is clear from table no.**4.5.16** and figure No.21 that all interaction means score and conclusion that the Science Rural male students got more score in Mental Health than other students. The highest mean score **19.75** was Science Rural male students.

4.6.1 The Respondents socio personal variables and their 3x2x2 factorial design for Integration of personality a part of mental health

Table No.4.6.1
The mean score for Independent variables on Integration of personality a part of Mental Health

Variables	A1(Arts faculty)		A2(Commerce faculty)		A3(Science faculty)	
C1 (Rural area)	B1 male students	B2 female students	B1 male students	B2 female students	B1 male students	B2 female students
	∑X=1178 MX=19.63 N=60	∑X=1184 MX=19.73 N=60	∑X=1222 MX=20.37 N=60	∑X=1206 MX=20.1 N=60	∑X=1244 MX=20.73 N=60	∑X=1196 MX=19.93 N=60
C2 (Urban area)	∑X=1190 MX=19.83 N=60	∑X=1195 MX=19.92 N=60	∑X=1224 MX=20.40 N=60	∑X=1210 MX=20.17 N=60	∑X=1129 MX=18.82 N=60	∑X=1102 MX=18.37 N=60

It could be seen from the table no.**4.6.1** the mean score for Independent variables on Integration of personality a part of Mental Health. The highest mean score was 20.73 of rural male Science students and the lowest mean score was 18.37 of urban female from Science faculty students.

Table 4.6.2
F calculation for Integration of personality a part of mental health
(3x2x2 factorial designed)

Sources of variance	Sum of square	d.f.	Mean square	F	Significance level
Ass (Types of faculty)	78.84	2	39.42	6.86	0.01
Bss (Sex)	11.36	1	11.36	1.98	N.S.
Css (Area)	34.79	1	34.79	6.05	0.05
ABss	11.82	2	5.49	1.03	N.S.
ACss	105.52	2	53.76	9.35	0.01
BCss	0.14	1	0.14	0.02	N.S.
ABCss	0.24	2	0.12	0.02	N.S
Wss	4069.35	708	5.75	-	-
Tss	4316.00	719	-	-	-

Significance levels df_1 0.05 = 3.85, 0.01= 6.66
df_2 0.05 = 3.00, 0.01= 4.62

The table no.**4.6.2** shows that F value of types of faculty variable was **6.86**, which was significance at **0.01** levels. The F value of sex variables was 1.98, which was not significance at **0.05** levels. The F value of Area variables was **6.05**, which was significance at **0.05** levels. The F value of Interaction to types of faculty and Sex variables was **1.03**, which was not significance at **0.05** levels. The F value of Interaction to types of faculty and Area variables was **9.35**, which was significance at **0.01** levels.

The F value of Interaction to Sex and Area variables was **0.02**, which was not significance at **0.05** levels. The F value of Interaction to types of faculty, Sex and Area variables was **0.021**.

Ho_{22}: There is no significance difference of Integration of personality a part of Mental Health based on types of faculty variable.

Table No. 4.6.3
The mean and F value for Types of faculty variable on Integration of personality a part of mental health

No.	Variables	N	Mean	F	Significance
1	Arts faculty students (A_1)	240	19.78		
2	Commerce faculty students(A_2)	240	20.26	**6.86**	**0.01**
3	Science faculty students(A3)	240	19.46		

Significance levels df_2 = 0.05=3.00 / 0.01=4.63

Table No. 4.6.4
L.S.D. values for Types of faculty variable on Integration of personality a part of mental health

Sr.No.	Pairs	Mean Diff.	Significance
1	A_1 vs. A_2	0.48	0.05
2	A_1 vs. A_3	0.32	N.S
3	A_2 vs. A_3	0.80	0.01

Sig. levels for L.S.D. 0.05=0.43 / 0.01=0.56

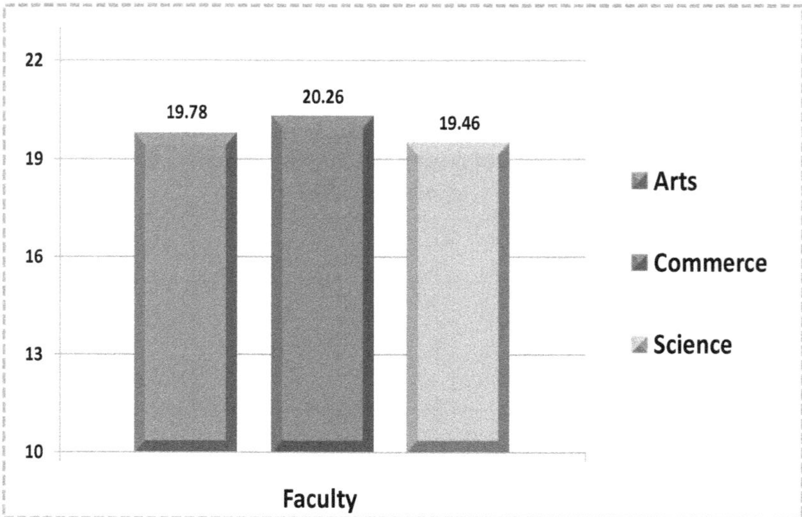

Figure No.22
Bar Chart of mean score of types of Faculty on Integration of personality a part of Mental Health

It is clear from the table no.**4.6.3** the mean score for the Arts faculty respondents were **19.78**, the mean score of Commerce faculty respondents were **20.26** and the mean score of Science faculty respondents were **19.46**. The F value for types of Faculty variable was **6.86** high was significant at 0.01 levels. Thus, Ho_{22} was rejected at 0.01 levels. So it can say that there was significant difference between types of Faculty on Integration of personality a part of Mental Health.

It could be seen from the table No.**4.6.4** and figure no.**22** that L.S.D. values for types of faculty on Integration of personality a part of Mental Health. The mean difference between Arts and Commerce faculty respondent was **0.48** which were significant at 0.05 levels. The mean difference between Arts and Science faculty respondent was **0.32**, which was not significant at 0.05 levels. The mean difference between Commerce and Science respondents was **0.80**, which was significant difference at 0.01 levels.

Ho23: There is no significance difference of Integration of personality a part of Mental Health based on Sex variables.

Table No 4.6.5
Mean score of Sex variables on Integration of personality a part of Mental Health

Variables	N	Mean score	F	Sig.
B_1 (Male)	360	19.97	**1.98**	**N.S.**
B_2 (Female)	360	19.70		

Significance levels df_2 =0.05=3.85 / 0.01=6.66

Table No. 4.6.6
L.S.D. values for Sex variable on Integration of personality a part of Mental Health

No.	Variables(Sex)	N	Mean diff.	Significance
1	B_1 (Male)	360	**0.27**	N.S.
2	B_2 (Female)	360		

Significance levels for L.S.D. =0.05=0.35 / 0.01=0.46

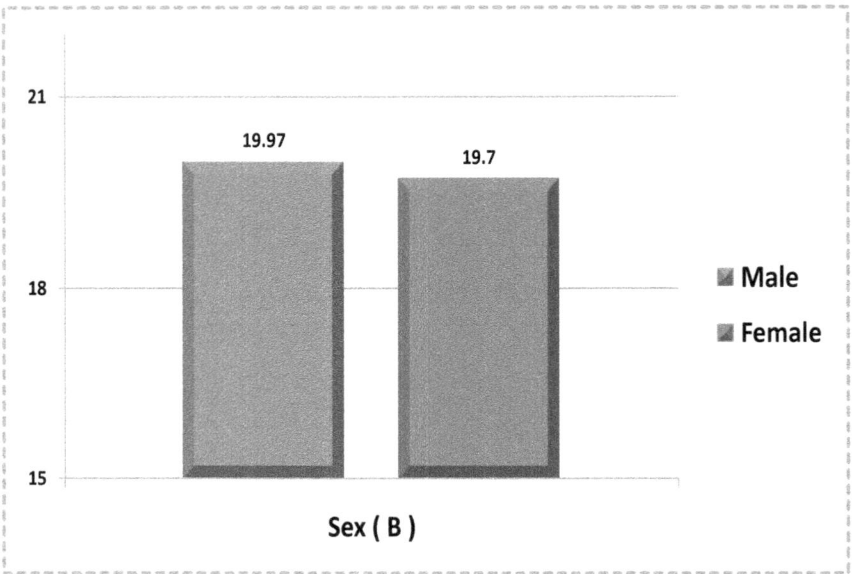

Figure No.23
Bar chart of mean score of sex variables on Integration of personality a part of Mental Health

It is observed from the table No. **4.6.5** that the mean for male students was **19.97** and the mean for Female students was **19.70**. The F value for sex variables was **1.98,** which was not significance at **0.05** levels. Hence, the **Ho_{23}** was not rejected and it could be said that there was significant mean difference between types of sex & their Integration of personality a part of Mental Health score. So it saw the result and said that the male students are more Integration of personality a part of Mental Health than female students. Hence it concluded that Integration types Mental Health was very affected factor for male students.

The table No. **4.6.6** and figure **No.23** point out the L.S.D. for Types of Sex variables on Integration types Mental Health that the mean different between Male and Female students on Integration types Mental Health was **0.27**, which was not Significance at **0.05** levels. Thus it concluded that the Male students are more Integration of personality a part of Mentally Healthy than Female students. Hence it concluded that Integration of personality a part of mental health was not very affected factor for Male students.

Ho_{24}: There is no significance difference on Integration of personality a part of Mental Health on Area variables.

Table No 4.6.7

Mean score and F value of Area variables on Integration of personality a part of mental health

Variables	N	Mean score	F	Sig.
C_1 (Rural)	360	20.01	**6.05**	**0.05**
C_2 (Urban)	360	19.61		

Significance levels df_2 =0.05=3.85 / 0.01=6.66

Table No. 4.6.8

L.S.D. values for Area variable on Integration of personality a part of Mental Health

No.	Variables(Area)	N	Mean diff.	Significance
1	Rural students (c_1)	360	**0.40**	**0.05**
2	Urban students (c_2)	360		

Significance levels for L.S.D. =0.05=0.35 / 0.01=0.46

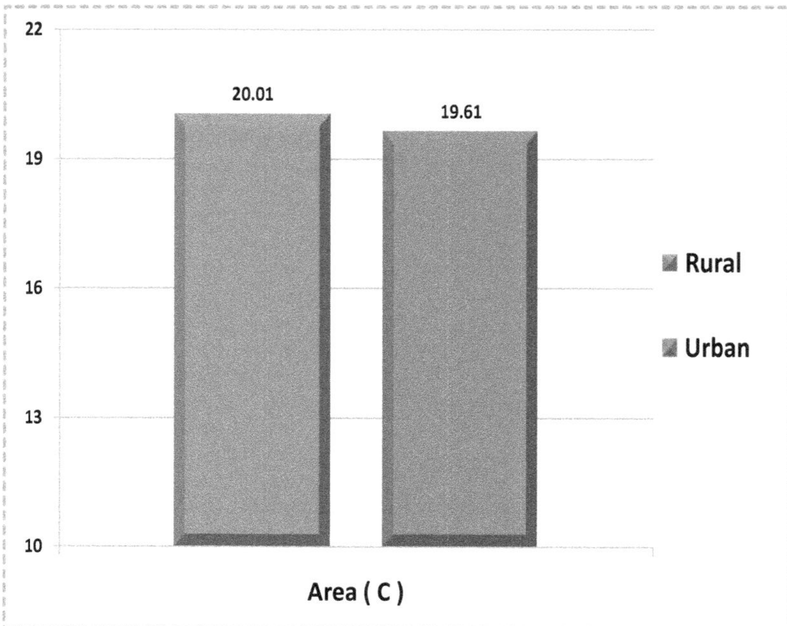

Figure No.24
Bar chart of mean score of Area variables of Integration of personality a part of mental health

It could be seen from the table No. **4.6.7** that the mean for rural students was **20.01** and the mean for urban students was **19.61**. The F value for **Area** variables was **6.05,** which was significance at **0.05** levels. Hence, the **Ho$_{24}$** was rejected and it could be said that there was significant mean difference between type of area & their Integration of personality a part of mental health score.

The table No. **4.6.8** and figure **No.24** indicated the L.S.D. for types of Area variables on Integration a part of mental health that the mean different between Rural and Urban students on Integration of personality a part of mental health was **6.05**, which was Significant at **0.05** levels. Thus it concluded that the rural students are more Integration type Mentally Healthy than Urban students. Hence it concluded that Integration a part of mental health was very affected factor for rural students.

Ho_{25}: There is no significance difference of Integration of personality a part of mental health based on Interaction for types of faculty and Sex variables.

Table No 4.6.9

Interaction F for types of faculty and Sex variables on Integration of personality a part of mental health

Variables	A_1 Arts students	A_2 commerce students	A_3 Science students	F	Sig.
B_1 Male students	**19.73**	**20.38**	**19.78**	**1.03**	**N.S.**
B_2 Female students	**19.83**	**20.13**	**19.15**		

Significance levels df2 =0.05=3.00 / 0.01=4.63

Table No 4.6.10

A L.S.D. Table for Interaction of Types of faculty and Sex variables on Integration of personality a part of mental health

Sr.N0.	Pairs	Mean Diff.	Significance
1	A_1B_1 vs. A_1B_2	0.10	N.S.
2	A_1B_1 vs. A_2B_1	0.65	0.05
3	A_1B_1 vs. A_2B_2	0.40	N.S.
4	A_1B_1 vs. A_3B_1	0.05	N.S.
5	A_1B_1 vs. A_3B_2	0.58	N.S.
6	A_1B_2 vs. A_2B_1	0.55	N.S.
7	A_1B_2 vs. A_2B_2	0.30	N.S.
8	A_1B_2 vs. A_3B_1	0.05	N.S.
9	A_1B_2 vs. A_3B_2	0.68	0.05
10	A_2B_1 vs. A_2B_2	0.25	N.S.
11	A_2B_1 vs. A_3B_1	0.60	N.S.
12	A_2B_1 vs. A_3B_2	1.23	0.01
13	A_2B_2 vs. A_3B_1	0.35	N.S.
14	A_2B_2 vs. A_3B_2	0.98	0.01
15	A_3B_1 vs. A_3B_2	0.63	0.05

Sig. levels for L.S.D. 0.05=0.61 / 0.01=0.79

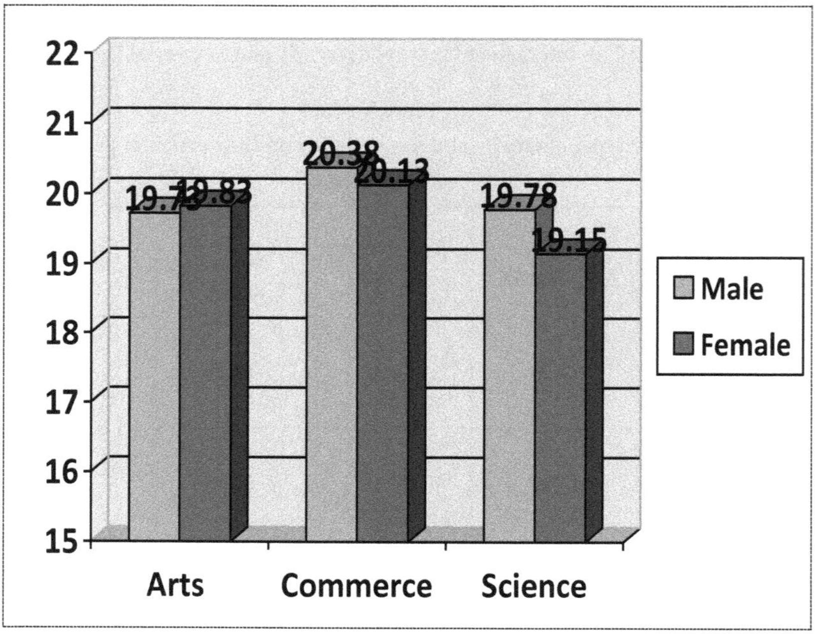

Figure No.25
Bar chart of mean score of Interaction of Types of faculty and Sex variables on Integration of personality a part of mental health

It is observed that the table No.**4.6.9** reveals the Interaction F for Type of faculty and Sex variables on Integration a part of mental health. The F value was **1.03**, which was not significance at **0.05** levels. Hence, the **Ho_{25}** was not rejected and it could be said that there was not significant mean difference between Types of faculty and sex variables & their Integration a part of mental health score.

The table no.**4.6.10** and figure **No.25** shows L.S.D. for interaction of types of faculty and sex variables on Integration a part of mental health. It shows the result and said that most of the pairs are significance at 0.05 or 0.01 levels. It also said that the highest mean score 20.37 was Commerce male students. The highest mean difference between A_2B_1 vs. A_3B_2 (Commerce male students Vs. Science female students) was **1.23**, it was big difference. The lowest mean difference between A_1B_2 vs. A_3B_1 (Arts female students Vs. Science male students) was **0.05** on Integration a part of mental health. Hence, all the result and concluded that either all variables (faculties and sex) are affected on Integration a part of mental health or Integration a part of mental health was affected them.

Ho_{26}: There is no significance difference of Integration of personality a part of mental health based on Interaction for types of faculty and Area variables.

Table No 4.6.11
Interaction F for types of faculty and Area variables on Integration of personality a part of mental health

Variables	A_1 Arts faculty students	A_2 Commerce faculty students	A_3 Science faculty students	F	Sig.
C_1 (Rural)	**18.18**	**20.23**	**20.33**	**9.35**	**0.01**
C_2 (Urban)	**18.71**	**20.28**	**18.60**		

Significance levels df2 =0.05=3.00 / 0.01=4.63

Table No 4.6.12
A L.S.D. Table for Interaction of Types of faculty and Area variables on Integration of personality a part of mental health

Sr.N0.	Pairs	Mean Diff.	Significance
1	A_1C_1 vs. A_1C_2	0.53	N.S.
2	A_1C_1 vs. A_2C_1	2.15	0.01
3	A_1C_1 vs. A_2C_2	2.10	0.01
4	A_1C_1 vs.A_3C_1	2.15	0.01
5	A_1C_1 vs.A_3C_2	0.42	N.S.
6	A_1C_2 vs. A_2C_1	1.52	0.01
7	A_1C_2 vs. A_2C_2	1.57	0.01
8	A_1C_2 vs. A_3C_1	1.62	0.01
9	A_1C_2 vs.A_3C_2	0.11	N.S.
10	A_2C_1 vs.A_2C_2	0.05	N.S.
11	A_2C_1 vs.A_3C_1	0.10	N.S.
12	A_2C_1 vs.A_3C_2	1.63	0.01
13	A_2C_2 vs.A_3C_1	0.05	N.S.
14	A_2C_2 vs.A_3C_2	1.68	0.01
15	A_3C_1 vs.A_3C_2	1.73	0.01

Sig. levels for L.S.D. 0.05=0.61 / 0.01=0.79

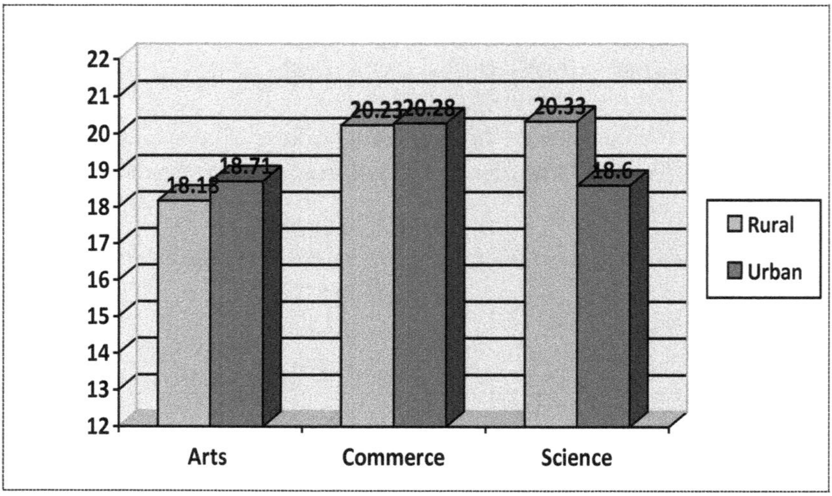

Figure No.26
Bar chart of interaction of Faculty and Area variables on Integration of personality a part of mental health

The table No.**4.6.11** indicated that the Interaction F for types of faculty and Area variables on Integration a part of mental health. The F value was **9.35**, which was significance at **0.01** levels. Hence, the **Ho_{26}** was rejected and it could be said that there was significant mean difference between types of faculty and area variables & their Integration a part of mental health score.

It could be seen from the no.**4.6.12** and figure **No.26** L.S.D. for interaction between the types of faculty and area variables on Integration a part of mental health. That it seen the result and said that the most of pairs significance at 0.05 or 0.01 levels. It also said the highest mean difference between A_1C_1 vs. A_2C_1 (Arts rural students Vs. Commerce rural students) was **2.15**, so we can said that it was big difference. The lowest mean difference between A_2C_2vs.A_3C_1 (Commerce urban students Vs. Science rural students) was **0.05** on Integration a part of mental health.

Ho_{27}: There is no significance difference of Integration of personality part of mental health based on for Sex variables and Area variables.

Table No 4.6.13

Interaction F for Sex variables and Area variables on Integration of personality part of mental health

Variables	B_1(Male students)	B_2 (Female students)	F	Sig.
C1 Rural students	20.24	19.92	**0.02**	**N.S.**
C2 Urban students	19.68	19.48		

Significance levels df_2 =0.05=3.85 / 0.01=6.66

Table No 4.6.14

A L.S.D. Table for Interaction of Sex and Area variables on Integration of personality part of mental health

Sr.N0.	Pairs	Mean Diff.	Significance
1	B_1C_1 vs. B_1C_2	0.56	0.05
2	B_1C_1 vs. B_2C_1	0.32	N.S.
3	B_1C_1 vs. B_2C_2	0.76	0.01
4	B_1C_2 vs.B_2C_1	0.24	N.S.
5	B_1C_2 vs. B_2C_2	0.20	N.S.
6	B_2C_1 vs. B_2C_2	0.44	N.S.

Sig. levels for L.S.D. 0.05=0.50 / 0.01=0.65

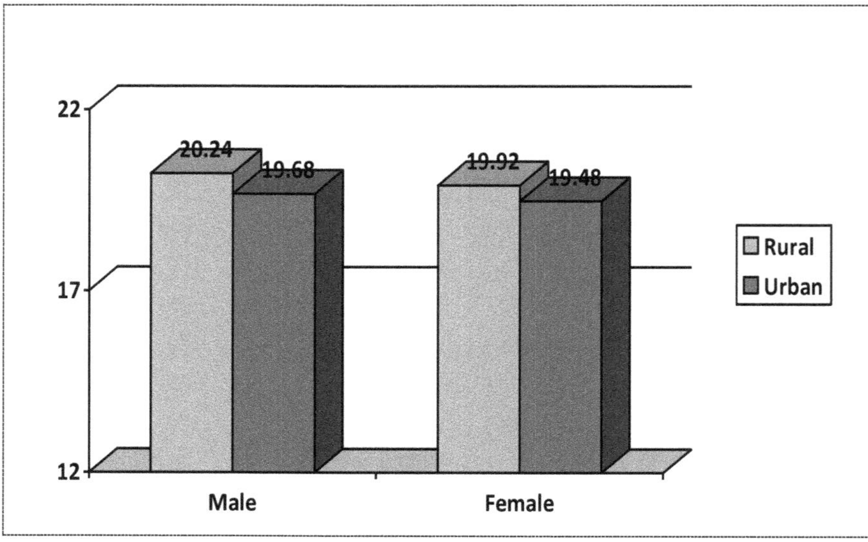

Figure No. 27
Bar chart of interaction of Sex and Area variables on Integration of personality part of mental health

The table No.**4.6.13** shows that the Interaction F for Sex variables and Area variables on Integration a part of mental health. F value was **0.02**, which was not significance at **0.05** levels. Hence, the **Ho_{26}** was not rejected at 0.05 levels and it could be said that there was no significant mean difference between Sex variables and Area variables & their Integration a part of mental health score.

It could be seen from the table **4.6.14** and figure **No.27** L.S.D. for interaction between the Sex variables and Area variables on Integration a part of mental health, that it seen the result and said that most of pairs are significance at 0.05 levels. It also said highest mean difference between B_1C_1vs. B_2C_2 (male rural students Vs. female urban students) was 0.76, so it was big difference. The lowest mean difference score between B_2C_1 vs. B_2C_2 (female rural students vs. female urban students) was 0.20 on Integration a part of mental health.

Ho_{28}: There is no significance difference of Integration of personality part of mental health based on Interaction for types of faculty, Sex and Area variables.

Table No 4.6.15

Interaction F for types of Faculty, Sex and Area variables on Integration of personality a part of mental health

variables	A_1 (Arts students)		A_2 (Commerce students)		A_3 (Science students)		F	Signi.
	B_1 male students	B_2 female students	B_1 male students	B_2 female students	B_1 male students	B_2 female students		
C_1	19.63	19.83	20.37	20.40	20.73	18.82	0.02	N.S.
C_2	19.73	19.92	20.10	20.17	19.93	18.37		

Significance levels df_1 =0.05=3.00 / 0.01=4.6

Table No 4.6.16

A L.S.D. Table for Interaction of types of faculty, Sex and Area variables on Integration of personality part of mental health

Sr.No.	Pairs	Mean Diff.	Significance
1	$A_1B_1C_1$ vs. $A_1B_1C_2$	0.10	N.S.
2	$A_1B_1C_1$ vs. $A_1B_2C_1$	0.20	N.S.
3	$A_1B_1C_1$ vs. $A_1B_2C_2$	0.29	N.S.
4	$A_1B_1C_1$ vs. $A_2B_1C_1$	0.74	N.S.
5	$A_1B_1C_1$ vs. $A_2B_1C_2$	0.47	N.S.
6	$A_1B_1C_1$ vs. $A_2B_2C_1$	0.77	N.S.
7	$A_1B_1C_1$ vs. $A_2B_2C_2$	0.54	N.S.
8	$A_1B_1C_1$ vs. $A_3B_1C_1$	1.10	0.05
9	$A_1B_1C_1$ vs. $A_3B_1C_2$	0.30	N.S.
10	$A_1B_1C_1$ vs. $A_3B_2C_1$	0.81	N.S.
11	$A_1B_1C_1$ vs. $A_3B_2C_2$	1.26	0.01
12	$A_1B_1C_2$ vs. $A_1B_2C_1$	0.10	N.S.
13	$A_1B_1C_2$ vs. $A_1B_2C_2$	0.19	N.S.
14	$A_1B_1C_2$ vs. $A_2B_1C_1$	0.64	N.S.

15	$A_1B_1C_2$ vs. $A_2B_1C_2$	0.37	N.S.
16	$A_1B_1C_2$ vs. $A_2B_2C_1$	0.67	N.S.
17	$A_1B_1C_2$ vs. $A_2B_2C_2$	0.44	N.S.
18	$A_1B_1C_2$ vs. $A_3B_1C_1$	1.00	0.05
19	$A_1B_1C_2$ vs. $A_3B_1C_2$	0.20	N.S.
20	$A_1B_1C_2$ vs. $A_3B_2C_1$	0.91	0.05
21	$A_1B_1C_2$ vs. $A_3B_2C_2$	1.36	0.01
22	$A_1B_2C_1$ vs. $A_1B_2C_2$	0.09	N.S.
23	$A_1B_2C_1$ vs. $A_2B_1C_1$	0.54	N.S.
24	$A_1B_2C_1$ vs. $A_2B_1C_2$	0.27	N.S.
25	$A_1B_2C_1$ vs. $A_2B_2C_1$	0.57	N.S.
26	$A_1B_2C_1$ vs. $A_2B_2C_2$	0.34	N.S.
27	$A_1B_2C_1$ vs. $A_3B_1C_1$	0.90	0.05
28	$A_1B_2C_1$ vs. $A_3B_1C_2$	0.10	N.S.
29	$A_1B_2C_1$ vs. $A_3B_2C_1$	1.01	0.05
30	$A_1B_2C_1$ vs. $A_3B_2C_2$	1.46	0.01
31	$A_1B_2C_2$ vs. $A_2B_1C_1$	0.45	N.S.
32	$A_1B_2C_2$ vs. $A_2B_1C_2$	0.18	N.S.
33	$A_1B_2C_2$ vs. $A_2B_2C_1$	0.48	N.S
34	$A_1B_2C_2$ vs. $A_2B_2C_2$	0.25	N.S.
35	$A_1B_2C_2$ vs. $A_3B_1C_1$	0.81	N.S.
36	$A_1B_2C_2$ vs. $A_3B_1C_2$	0.01	N.S.
37	$A_1B_2C_2$ vs. $A_3B_2C_1$	1.10	0.5
38	$A_1B_2C_2$ vs. $A_3B_2C_2$	1.55	0.01
39	$A_2B_1C_1$ vs. $A_2B_1C_2$	0.27	N.S.
40	$A_2B_1C_1$ vs. $A_2B_2C_1$	0.03	N.S.
41	$A_2B_1C_1$ vs. $A_2B_2C_2$	0.20	N.S.
42	$A_2B_1C_1$ vs. $A_3B_1C_1$	0.36	N.S.
43	$A_2B_1C_1$ vs. $A_3B_1C_2$	0.44	N.S.
44	$A_2B_1C_1$ vs. $A_3B_2C_1$	1.55	0.01
45	$A_2B_1C_1$ vs. $A_3B_2C_2$	2.00	0.01
46	$A_2B_1C_2$ vs. $A_2B_2C_1$	0.30	N.S.
47	$A_2B_1C_2$ vs. $A_2B_2C_2$	0.07	N.S.

48	$A_2B_1C_2$ vs. $A_3B_1C_1$	0.63	N.S.
49	$A_2B_1C_2$ vs. $A_3B_1C_2$	0.17	N.S.
50	$A_2B_1C_2$ vs. $A_3B_2C_1$	1.28	0.01
51	$A_2B_1C_2$ vs. $A_3B_2C_2$	1.73	0.01
52	$A_2B_2C_1$ vs. $A_2B_2C_2$	0.23	N.S.
53	$A_2B_2C_1$ vs. $A_3B_1C_1$	0.33	N.S.
54	$A_2B_2C_1$ vs. $A_3B_1C_2$	0.47	N.S.
55	$A_2B_2C_1$ vs. $A_3B_2C_1$	1.58	0.01
56	$A_2B_2C_1$ vs. $A_3B_2C_2$	2.03	0.01
57	$A_2B_2C_2$ vs. $A_3B_1C_1$	0.56	N.S.
58	$A_2B_2C_2$ vs. $A_3B_1C_2$	0.24	N.S.
59	$A_2B_2C_2$ vs. $A_3B_2C_1$	1.35	0.01
60	$A_2B_2C_2$ vs. $A_3B_2C_2$	1.80	0.01
61	$A_3B_1C_1$ vs. $A_3B_1C_2$	0.80	N.S.
62	$A_3B_1C_1$ vs. $A_3B_2C_1$	1.91	0.01
63	$A_3B_1C_1$ vs. $A_3B_2C_2$	2.36	0.01
64	$A_3B_1C_2$ vs. $A_3B_2C_1$	1.11	0.01
65	$A_3B_1C_2$vs. $A_3B_2C_2$	1.56	0.01
66	$A_3B_2C_1$ vs. $A_3B_2C_2$	0.45	N.S.

Sig. levels for L.S.D. 0.05=0.86 / 0.01=1.13

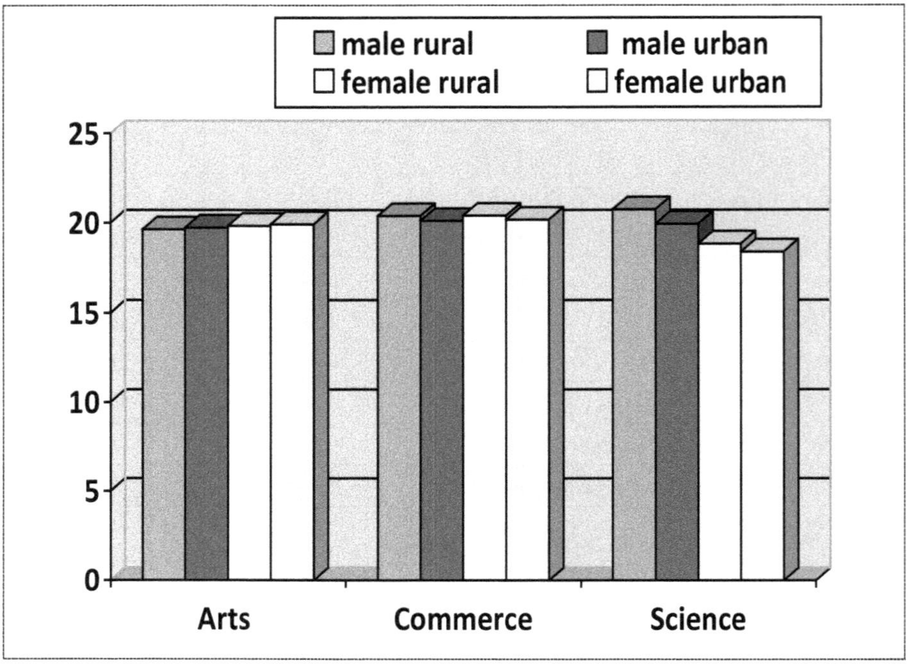

Figure No.28
The bar chart of interaction between the types of faculty, sex and area variables on Integration a part of mental health

The table No.**4.6.15** indicated that the Interaction F for Sex and Area variables on Perception of reality types Mental Health. F value was **0.02,** which was not significance at **0.05** levels. Hence, the **Ho_{28}** was not rejected and it could be said that there was no significant mean difference between sex and area variables & their Integration a part of mental health score.

It could be seen the all interaction means score and conclusion that the Science Rural male students got more score Integration a part of mental health than other students. The highest mean score **20.73** was Science Rural male students.

The tables No.**4.6.16** and figure No.**28** point out that most of pairs were not significant at 0.05 levels. The high mean different was 2.36 ($A_3B_1C_1$ vs. $A_3B_2C_1$) and lowest score was 0.01($A_1B_2C_2$ vs. $A_3B_1C_1$).

4.7.1 The Respondents socio personal variables and their 3x2x2 factorial design for Positive self-evolution a part of mental health

Table No.4.7.1

The mean score for Independent variables on Positive self-evolution a part of mental health

Variables	A1(Arts faculty)		A2(Commerce faculty)		A3(Science faculty)	
C1 (Rural area)	B1 male students	B2 female students	B1 male students	B2 female students	B1 male students	B2 female students
	ΣX=1126 MX=18.77 N=60	ΣX=1094 MX=18.23 N=60	ΣX=1161 MX=19.35 N=60	ΣX=1128 MX=18.8 N=60	ΣX=1179 MX=19.65 N=60	ΣX=1155 MX=19.25 N=60
C2 (Urban area)	ΣX=1147 MX=19.12 N=60	ΣX=1112 MX=18.53 N=60	ΣX=1145 MX=19.08 N=60	ΣX=1098 MX=18.3 N=60	ΣX=1103 MX=18.38 N=60	ΣX=1071 MX=17.85 N=60

It has seen the table no.4.63 the mean score for Independent variables on Positive self-evolution a part of mental health. The highest mean score was 19.65 of rural male Science students and the lowest mean score was 17.85 of urban female from Science faculty students.

Table 4.7.2
F calculation for Positive self-evolution a part of mental health
(3x2x2 factorial designed)

Sources of variance	Sum of square	d.f.	Mean square	F	Significance level
Ass (Types of faculty)	5.80	2	2.90	0.38	N.S.
Bss (Sex)	56.36	1	56.36	7.36	0.01
Css (Area)	37.78	1	37.78	4.93	0.01
ABss	1.29	2	0.64	0.08	N.S.
ACss	82.40	2	41.20	5.38	0.05
BCss	0.60	1	0.60	0.07	N.S.
ABCss	0.32	2	0.158	0.02	N.S.
Wss	5425.93	708	7.66	-	-
Tss	5612.99	719	-	-	-

Significance levels df_1 0.05 = 3.85, 0.01= 6.66
df_2 0.05 = 3.00, 0.01= 4.63

It has seen the table no.**4.7.2** that F value of types of faculty variable was **0.38**, which was not significance at **0.05** levels. The F value of sex variables was 7.36, which was significance at **0.01** levels. The F value of Area variables was **4.93**, which was significance at **0.01** levels. The F value of Interaction to types of faculty and Sex variables was **0.08**, which was not significance at **0.05** levels. The F value of Interaction to types of faculty and Area variables was **5.38**, which was significance at **0.05** levels.

The F value of Interaction to Sex and Area variables was **0.07**, which was not significance at **0.05** levels. The F value of Interaction to types of faculty, Sex and Area variables was **0.021**, which was not significance at **0.05** levels.

Ho_{22}: There is no significance difference of Positive self-evolution a part of mental health based on type of faculty variable.

Table No. 4.7.3
The mean and F value for Types of faculty variable on Positive self-evolution a part of mental health

No.	Variables	N	Mean	F	Significance
1	Arts faculty students (A_1)	240	18.67	**0.38**	**N.S.**
2	Commerce faculty students(A_2)	240	18.88		
3	Science faculty students(A3)	240	18.78		

Significance levels df_2 = 0.05=3.00 / 0.01=4.63

Table No. 4.7.4
L.S.D. values for Types of faculty variable on Positive self-evolution a part of mental health

Sr.No.	Pairs	Mean Diff.	Significance
1	A_1 vs. A_2	0.21	N.S.
2	A_1 vs. A_3	0.11	N.S.
3	A_2 vs. A_3	0.10	N.S.

Sig. levels for L.S.D. 0.05=0.50 / 0.01=0.65

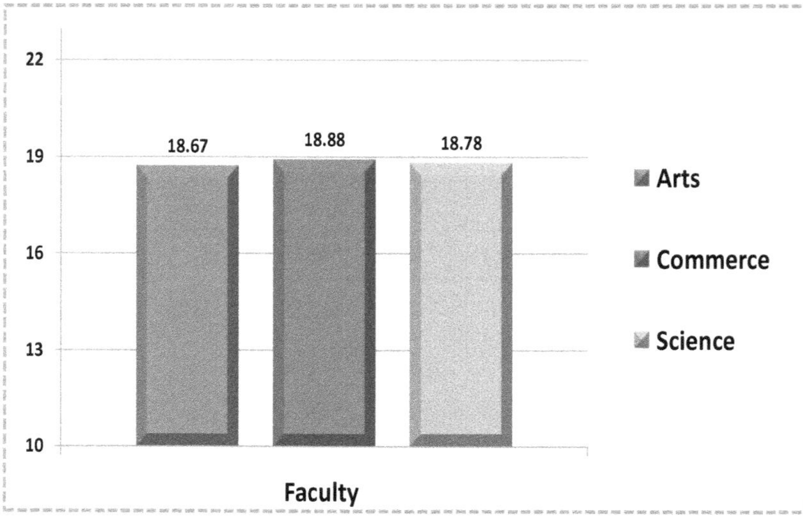

Figure No.29
Bar Char of mean score of types of Faculty on Positive self-evolution a part of mental health

It is observed from the table no.**4.7.3** the mean score for the Arts faculty respondents were **18.67**, the mean score of Commerce faculty respondents were **18.88** and the mean score of Science faculty respondents were **18.78**. The F value for types of Faculty variable was **0.38** which was not significant at 0.05 levels. Thus, Ho_{29} was not rejected at 0.05 levels. So it can say that there was no significant difference between types of Faculty on Positive self-evolution a part of mental health.

The table No.**4.7.4** and figure no.**29** indicated L.S.D. values for types of faculty on Positive self-evolution a part of mental health. The mean difference between Arts and Commerce faculty respondent was **0.21** which were not significant at 0.05 levels. The mean difference between Arts and Science faculty respondent was **0.11**, which was not significant at 0.05 levels. The mean difference between Commerce and Science respondents was 0.10, which was not significant difference at 0.05 levels.

Ho30: **There is no significance difference of Positive self-evolution a part of mental health based on Sex variables.**

Table No 4.7.5
Mean score of Sex variables on Positive self-evolution a part of mental health

Variables	N	Mean score	F	Sig.
B_1 (Male)	360	19.06	**7.36**	**0.01**
B_2 (Female)	360	18.49		

Significance levels df_2 =0.05=3.85 / 0.01=6.66

Table No. 4.7.6
L.S.D. values for Sex variable on Positive self-evolution a part of mental health

No.	Variables(Sex)	N	Mean diff.	Significance
1	B_1 (Male)	360	**0.57**	0.01
2	B_2 (Female)	360		

Significance levels for L.S.D. =0.05=0.35 / 0.01=0.46

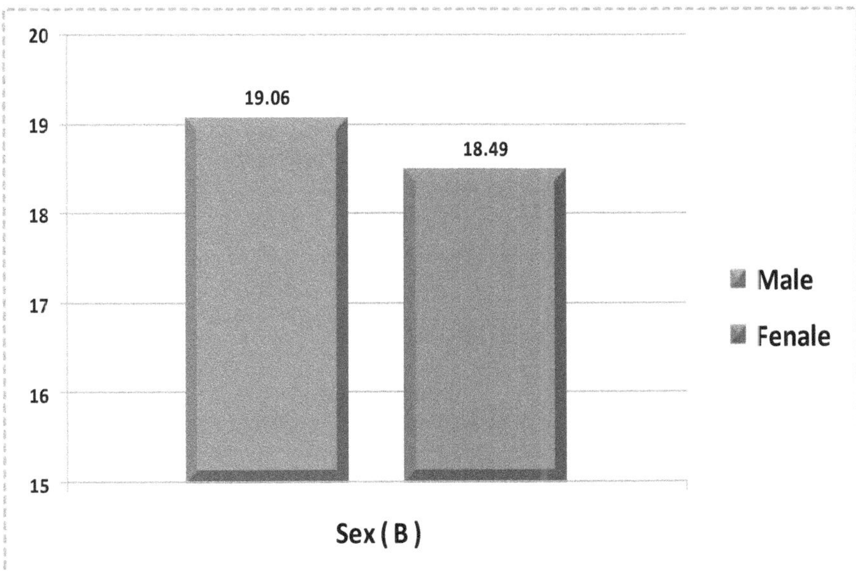

Figure No.30
Bar chart of mean score of sex variables on Positive self-evolution a part of mental health

It is observed from the table No. **4.7.5** that the mean for male students was **19.07** and the mean for Female students was **18.49**. The F value for sex variables was **7.36,** which was significance at **0.01** levels. Hence, the **Ho_{30}** was rejected and it could be said that there was significant mean difference between types of sex & their Positive self-evolution a part of mental health score. So it saw the result and said that the male students are more Positive self-evolution a part of mental health than female students. Hence it concluded that Positive self-evolution a part of mental health was very affected factor for male students.

It could be seen from the table No. **4.7.6** and figure **No.30** the L.S.D. for Types of Sex variables on Positive self-evolution a part of mental health that the mean different between Male and Female students on Positive self-evolution a part of mental health was **0.57**, which was Significance at **0.01** levels. Thus it concluded that the Male students are more Positive self-evolution type Mentally Healthy than Female students. Hence it concluded that Positive self-evolution a part of mental health was very affected factor for Male students.

Ho_{31}: There is no significance difference of Positive self-evolution a part of mental health on Area variables.

Table No 4.7.7
Mean score and F value of Area variables on Positive self-evolution a part of mental health

Variables	N	Mean score	F	Sig.
C_1 (Rural)	360	19.01	**4.93**	**0.05**
C_2 (Urban)	360	18.55		

Significance levels df_2 =0.05=3.85 / 0.01=6.66

Table No. 4.7.8
L.S.D. values for Area variable on Positive self-evolution a part of mental health

No.	Variables(Area)	N	Mean diff.	Significance
1	Rural students (c_1)	360	**0.46**	**0.05**
2	Urban students (c_2)	360		

Significance levels for L.S.D. =0.05=0.40 / 0.01=0.53

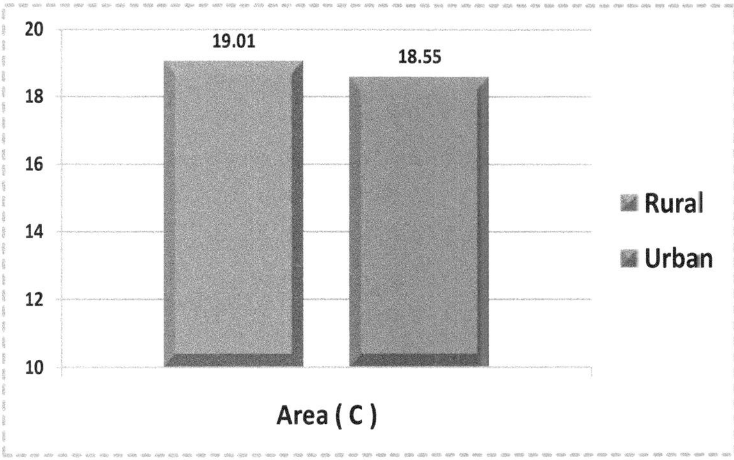

Figure No.31
Bar chart of mean score of Area variables of Positive self-evolution a part of mental health

The table No. **4.7.7** shows that the mean for rural students was **19.01** and the mean for urban students was **18.55**. The F value for **Area** variables was **4.93,** which was significance at **0.05** levels. Hence, the **Ho$_{31}$** was rejected and it could be said that there was significant mean difference between type of area & their Positive self-evolution a part of mental health score.

It could be seen from the table No. **4.7.8** and figure **No.31** the L.S.D. for types of Area variables on Positive self-evolution a part of mental health that the mean different between Rural and Urban students on Positive self-evolution a part of mental health was 4.93, which was Significant at **0.05** levels. Thus it concluded that the rural students are more Positive self-evolution type Mentally Healthy than Urban students. Hence it concluded that Positive self-evolution a part of mental health was very affected factor for Male students.

H_{o32}: There is no significance difference of Positive self-evolution a part of mental health based on Interaction for type of faculty and Sex variables.

Table No 4.7.9

Interaction F for types of faculty and Sex variables on Positive self-evolution a part of mental health

Variables	A_1 Arts students	A_2 commerce students	A_3 Science students	F	Sig.
B_1 Male students	**18.94**	**19.22**	**19.02**	**0.08**	**N.S.**
B_2 Female students	**18.38**	**18.55**	**18.55**		

Significance levels df2 =0.05=3.00 / 0.01=4.63

Table No 4.7.10

A L.S.D. Table for Interaction of Types of faculty and Sex variables on Positive self-evolution a part of mental health

Sr.No.	Pairs	Mean Diff.	Significance
1	A_1B_1 vs. A_1B_2	0.56	N.S.
2	A_1B_1 vs. A_2B_1	0.28	N.S.
3	A_1B_1 vs. A_2B_2	0.39	N.S.
4	A_1B_1 vs.A_3B_1	0.08	N.S.
5	A_1B_1 vs.A_3B_2	0.39	N.S.
6	A_1B_2 vs. A_2B_1	0.84	0.05
7	A_1B_2 vs. A_2B_2	0.17	N.S.
8	A_1B_2 vs. A_3B_1	0.64	N.S.
9	A_1B_2 vs.A_3B_2	0.17	N.S.
10	A_2B_1 vs.A_2B_2	0.67	N.S.
11	A_2B_1 vs.A_3B_1	0.20	N.S.
12	A_2B_1 vs.A_3B_2	067	N.S.
13	A_2B_2 vs.A_3B_1	0.47	N.S.
14	A_2B_2 vs.A_3B_2	0.00	N.S.
15	A_3B_1 vs.A_3B_2	0.47	N.S.

Sig. levels for L.S.D. 0.05=0.71/ 0.01=0.92

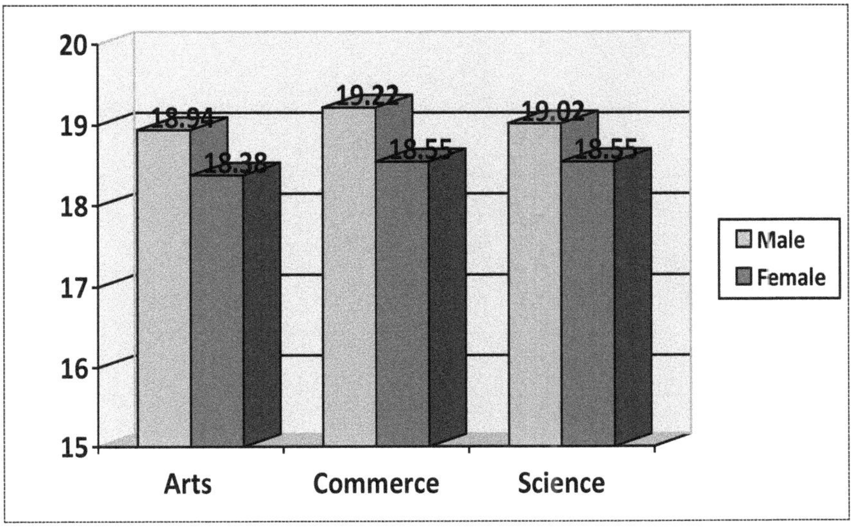

Figure No.32
Bar chart of mean score of Interaction of Types of faculty and Sex variables on Positive self-evolution a part of mental health

The table No.**4.7.9** indicated that the Interaction F for Type of faculty and Sex variables on Integration a part of mental health. The F value was **0.08**, which was not significance at **0.05** levels. Hence, the **Ho_{32}** was not rejected and it could be said that there was not significant mean difference between Types of faculty and sex variables & their Positive self-evolution a part of mental health score.

It was clear from the table no.**4.7.10** and figure**No.32** L.S.D. for interaction of types of faculty and sex variables **on** Positive self-evolution a part of mental health. The result said that most of the pairs are not significance at 0.05 or 0.01 levels. It also said that the highest mean score 19.22 was Commerce male students. The highest mean difference between A_1B_2 vs. A_3B_2 (Arts female students Vs. Science female students) was **0.84**, so it also said that it was big difference. The lowest mean difference between A_1B_2 vs. A_3B_1 (Arts female students Vs. Science male students) was **0.00** on Positive self-evolution a part of mental health. Hence, it sees all the result and concluded that either all variables (faculties and sex) are affected on Positive self-evolution a part of mental health or Positive self-evolution a part of mental health was affected them.

Ho_{33}: There is no significance difference of Positive self-evolution a part of mental health based on Interaction for types of faculty and Area variables.

Table No 4.7.11
Interaction F for types of faculty and Area variables on Positive self-evolution a part of mental health

Variables	A_1 (Arts faculty students)	A_2 (Commerce faculty students)	A_3 (Science faculty students)	F	Sig.
C_1 (Rural)	**18.5**	**19.08**	**19.45**	**5.38**	**0.01**
C_2 (Urban)	**18.83**	**18.69**	**18.12**		

Significance levels df2 =0.05=3.00 / 0.01=4.63

Table No 4.7.12
A L.S.D. Table for Interaction of Types of faculty and Area variables on Positive self-evolution a part of mental health

Sr.N0.	Pairs	Mean Diff.	Significance
1	A_1C_1 vs. A_1C_2	0.33	N.S.
2	A_1C_1 vs. A_2C_1	0.58	N.S.
3	A_1C_1 vs. A_2C_2	0.19	N.S.
4	A_1C_1 vs.A_3C_1	0.95	0.01
5	A_1C_1 vs.A_3C_2	0.38	N.S.
6	A_1C_2 vs. A_2C_1	0.25	N.S.
7	A_1C_2 vs. A_2C_2	0.14	N.S.
8	A_1C_2 vs. A_3C_1	0.62	N.S.
9	A_1C_2 vs.A_3C_2	0.71	0.05
10	A_2C_1 vs.A_2C_2	0.39	N.S.
11	A_2C_1 vs.A_3C_1	0.37	N.S.
12	A_2C_1 vs.A_3C_2	0.96	0.01
13	A_2C_2 vs.A_3C_1	0.76	0.05
14	A_2C_2 vs.A_3C_2	0.57	N.S.
15	A_3C_1 vs.A_3C_2	1.33	0.01

Sig. levels for L.S.D. 0.05=0.71 / 0.01=0.92

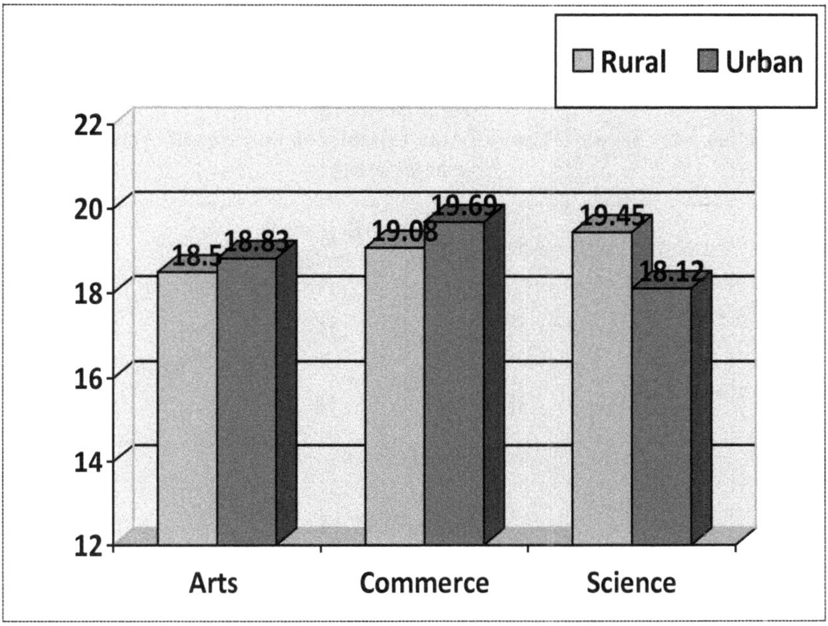

Figure No.33
Bar chart of interaction of Faculty and Area variables on Positive self-evolution a part of mental health

The table No.**4.7.11** points out that the Interaction F for types of faculty and Area variables on Positive self-evolution a part of mental health. The F value was **9.35**, which was significance at **0.01** levels. Hence, the **Ho$_{33}$** was rejected and it could be said that there was significant mean difference between types of faculty and area variables & their Positive self-evolution a part of mental health score.

It is clear from the table no.**4.7.12** and figure**No.33** L.S.D. for interaction between the types of faculty and area variables on Positive self-evolution a part of mental health. That it seen the result and said that the most of pairs significance at 0.05 or 0.01 levels. It also said the highest mean difference between A_2C_1 vs.A_3C_2 (Commerce rural students Vs. Science urban students) was **1.33**, so we can said that it was big difference. The lowest mean difference between A_1C_2vs.A_2C_1 (Arts urban students Vs. Commerce rural students) was **0.25** on Positive self-evolution a part of mental health.

Ho_{34}: There is no significance difference of Positive self-evolution a part of mental health based on for Sex variables and Area variables.

Table No 4.7.13
Interaction F for Sex variables and Area variables on Positive self-evolution a part of mental health

Variables	B_1(Male students)	B_2 (Female students)	F	Sig.
Rural students (C_1)	19.25	18.76	**0.078**	**N.S.**
Urban students (C_2)	18.86	18.23		

Significance levels df_2 =0.05=3.85/ 0.01=6.66

Table No 4.7.14
A L.S.D. Table for Interaction of Sex and Area variables on Positive self-evolution a part of mental health

Sr.N0.	Pairs	Mean Diff.	Significance
1	B_1C_1 vs. B_1C_2	0.39	N.S.
2	B_1C_1 vs. B_2C_1	0.49	N.S.
3	B_1C_1 vs. B_2C_2	1.02	0.01
4	B_1C_2 vs. B_2C_1	0.10	N.S.
5	B_1C_2 vs. B_2C_2	0.63	0.05
6	B_2C_1 vs. B_2C_2	0.53	N.S.

Sig. levels for L.S.D. 0.05=0.57 / 0.01=0.74

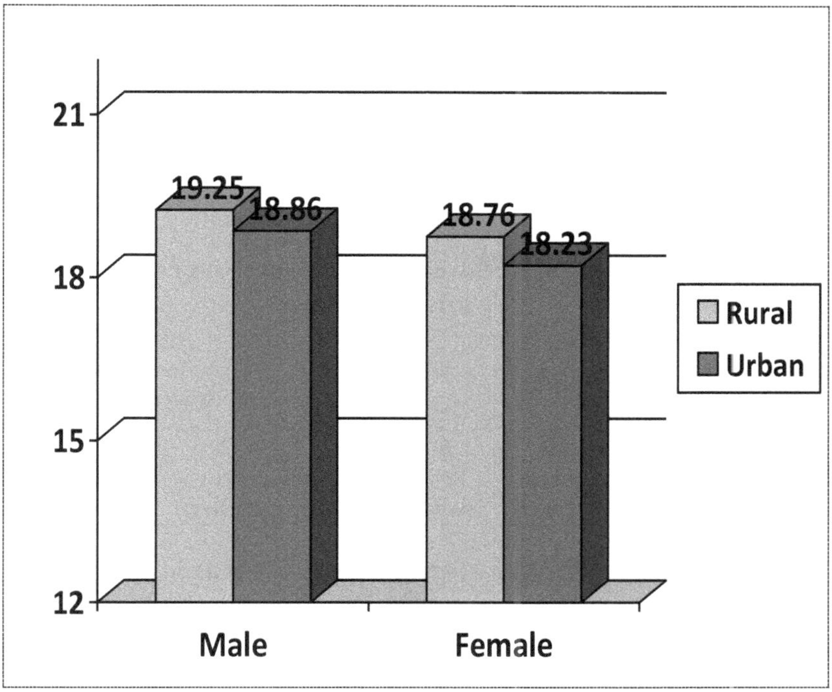

Figure No. 34
Bar chart of interaction of Sex and Area variables on Positive self-evolution a part of mental health

It has seen from the table No.**4.7.13** that the Interaction F for Sex variables and Area variables on Positive self-evolution a part of mental health. F value was **0.078**, which was not significance at **0.05** levels. Hence, the **Ho_{34}** was not rejected at 0.05 levels and it could be said that there was no significant mean difference between Sex variables and Area variables & their Positive self-evolution a part of mental health score.

It is clear from the table **4.7.14** and figure **No.34** L.S.D. for interaction between the Sex variables and Area variables on Positive self-evolution a part of mental health, that it seen the result and said that most of pairs are significance at 0.05 levels. It also said highest mean difference between B_1C_1vs. B_2C_2 (male rural students Vs. female urban students) was 1.02, so it said that it was big difference. The lowest mean difference score between B_2C_1 vs.

B_2C_2 (female rural students vs. female urban students) was 0.10 on Positive self-evolution a part of mental health.

Ho_{35}: There is no significance difference of Positive self-evolution a part of mental health based on Interaction for types of faculty, Sex and Area variables.

Table No 4.7.15
Interaction F for types of Faculty, Sex and Area variables on Positive self-evolution a part of mental health

variables	A_1(Arts students)		A_2(Commerce students)		A_3(Science students)		F	Sig.
	B_1 male students	B_2 female students	B_1 male students	B_2 female students	B_1 male students	B_2 female students		
C_1	18.77	18.23	19.35	18.80	19.65	19.25	0.02	N.S.
C_2	19.12	18.53	19.80	18.30	18.38	17.85		

Significance levels df_1 =0.05=3.00 / 0.01=4.63

Table No 4.7.16
A L.S.D. Table for Interaction of types of faculty, Sex and Area variables on Positive self-evolution a part of mental health

Sr.N0.	Pairs	Mean Diff.	Significance
1	$A_1B_1C_1$ vs. $A_1B_1C_2$	0.35	N.S.
2	$A_1B_1C_1$ vs. $A_1B_2C_1$	0.54	N.S.
3	$A_1B_1C_1$ vs. $A_1B_2C_2$	0.24	N.S.
4	$A_1B_1C_1$ vs. $A_2B_1C_1$	0.58	N.S.
5	$A_1B_1C_1$ vs. $A_2B_1C_2$	1.03	0.01
6	$A_1B_1C_1$ vs. $A_2B_2C_1$	0.03	N.S.
7	$A_1B_1C_1$ vs. $A_2B_2C_2$	0.47	N.S.
8	$A_1B_1C_1$ vs. $A_3B_1C_1$	0.88	N.S.
9	$A_1B_1C_1$ vs. $A_3B_1C_2$	0.39	N.S.
10	$A_1B_1C_1$ vs. $A_3B_2C_1$	0.48	N.S.
11	$A_1B_1C_1$ vs. $A_3B_2C_2$	0.92	N.S.

12	$A_1B_1C_2$ vs. $A_1B_2C_1$	0.89	N.S.
13	$A_1B_1C_2$ vs. $A_1B_2C_2$	0.59	N.S.
14	$A_1B_1C_2$ vs. $A_2B_1C_1$	0.23	N.S.
15	$A_1B_1C_2$ vs. $A_2B_1C_2$	0.68	N.S.
16	$A_1B_1C_2$ vs. $A_2B_2C_1$	0.32	N.S.
17	$A_1B_1C_2$ vs. $A_2B_2C_2$	0.82	N.S.
18	$A_1B_1C_2$ vs. $A_3B_1C_1$	0.53	N.S.
19	$A_1B_1C_2$ vs. $A_3B_1C_2$	0.74	N.S.
20	$A_1B_1C_2$ vs. $A_3B_2C_1$	0.13	N.S.
21	$A_1B_1C_2$ vs. $A_3B_2C_2$	1.27	0.05
22	$A_1B_2C_1$ vs. $A_1B_2C_2$	0.30	N.S.
23	$A_1B_2C_1$ vs. $A_2B_1C_1$	1.12	0.05
24	$A_1B_2C_1$ vs. $A_2B_1C_2$	1.57	0.01
25	$A_1B_2C_1$ vs. $A_2B_2C_1$	0.57	N.S.
26	$A_1B_2C_1$ vs. $A_2B_2C_2$	0.07	N.S.
27	$A_1B_2C_1$ vs. $A_3B_1C_1$	1.42	0.01
28	$A_1B_2C_1$ vs. $A_3B_1C_2$	0.15	N.S.
29	$A_1B_2C_1$ vs. $A_3B_2C_1$	1.02	0.05
30	$A_1B_2C_1$ vs. $A_3B_2C_2$	0.38	N.S.
31	$A_1B_2C_2$ vs. $A_2B_1C_1$	0.82	N.S.
32	$A_1B_2C_2$ vs. $A_2B_1C_2$	1.27	0.05
33	$A_1B_2C_2$ vs. $A_2B_2C_1$	0.27	N.S.
34	$A_1B_2C_2$ vs. $A_2B_2C_2$	0.23	N.S.
35	$A_1B_2C_2$ vs. $A_3B_1C_1$	1.12	0.05
36	$A_1B_2C_2$ vs. $A_3B_1C_2$	0.15	N.S.
37	$A_1B_2C_2$ vs. $A_3B_2C_1$	0.72	N.S.
38	$A_1B_2C_2$ vs. $A_3B_2C_2$	0.68	N.S.
39	$A_2B_1C_1$ vs. $A_2B_1C_2$	0.45	N.S.
40	$A_2B_1C_1$ vs. $A_2B_2C_1$	0.55	N.S.
41	$A_2B_1C_1$ vs. $A_2B_2C_2$	1.05	0.05
42	$A_2B_1C_1$ vs. $A_3B_1C_1$	0.30	N.S.
43	$A_2B_1C_1$ vs. $A_3B_1C_2$	0.97	N.S.
44	$A_2B_1C_1$ vs. $A_3B_2C_1$	0.10	N.S.

45	$A_2B_1C_1$ vs. $A_3B_2C_2$	1.50	0.01
46	$A_2B_1C_2$ vs. $A_2B_2C_1$	1.00	0.05
47	$A_2B_1C_2$ vs. $A_2B_2C_2$	1.50	0.01
48	$A_2B_1C_2$ vs. $A_3B_1C_1$	0.15	N.S.
49	$A_2B_1C_2$ vs. $A_3B_1C_2$	1.42	0.01
50	$A_2B_1C_2$ vs. $A_3B_2C_1$	0.55	N.S.
51	$A_2B_1C_2$ vs. $A_3B_2C_2$	1.95	0.01
52	$A_2B_2C_1$ vs. $A_2B_2C_2$	0.50	N.S.
53	$A_2B_2C_1$ vs. $A_3B_1C_1$	0.85	N.S.
54	$A_2B_2C_1$ vs. $A_3B_1C_2$	0.42	N.S.
55	$A_2B_2C_1$ vs. $A_3B_2C_1$	0.45	N.S.
56	$A_2B_2C_1$ vs. $A_3B_2C_2$	0.95	N.S.
57	$A_2B_2C_2$ vs. $A_3B_1C_1$	1.35	0.01
58	$A_2B_2C_2$ vs. $A_3B_1C_2$	0.08	N.S.
59	$A_2B_2C_2$ vs. $A_3B_2C_1$	0.95	N.S.
60	$A_2B_2C_2$ vs. $A_3B_2C_2$	0.45	N.S.
61	$A_3B_1C_1$ vs. $A_3B_1C_2$	1.27	0.05
62	$A_3B_1C_1$ vs. $A_3B_2C_1$	0.40	N.S.
63	$A_3B_1C_1$ vs. $A_3B_2C_2$	1.80	0.01
64	$A_3B_1C_2$ vs. $A_3B_2C_1$	0.87	N.S.
65	$A_3B_1C_2$vs. $A_3B_2C_2$	0.53	N.S.
66	$A_3B_2C_1$ vs. $A_3B_2C_2$	1.40	0.01

Sig. levels for L.S.D. 0.05=1.00 / 0.01=1.31

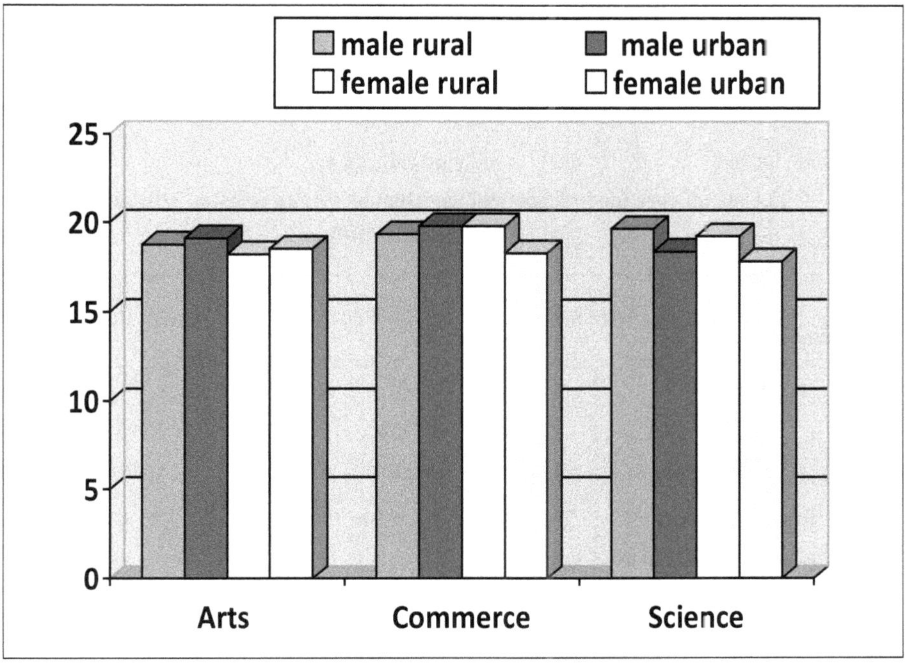

Figure No.35
Bar chart of interaction of the types of faculty, Sex and Area variables on Positive self-evolution a part of mental health

It is clear from the table No.**4.7.15** that the Interaction F for types of Faculty, Sex variables and Area variables on Positive self-evolution a part of mental health. F value was **0.021**, which was not significance at **0.05** levels. Hence, the **Ho_{35}** was not rejected at 0.05 levels and it could be said that there was no significant mean difference between Sex variables and Area variables & their Positive self-evolution a part of mental health score.

The table **4.7.16 and figure no.35** indicated the L.S.D. for interaction between the Types of faculty, Sex variables and Area variables on Positive self-evolution a part of mental health, that it seen the result and said that most of pairs are significance at 0.05 levels. It also said highest mean difference between B_1C_1vs. B_2C_2 (male rural students vs. female urban students) was **1.95**, so it said that it was big difference. The lowest mean difference score between B_2C_1 vs. B_2C_2 (female rural students vs. female urban students) was **0.10** on Positive self-evolution a part of mental health.

4.8.1 The Respondents socio personal variables and their 3x2x2 factorial design for Group oriented attitudes a part of mental health

Table No.4.8.1
The mean score for Independent variables on Group oriented attitudes a part of mental health

Variables	A1(Arts faculty)		A2(Commerce faculty)		A3(Science faculty)	
	B1 male students	B2 female students	B1 male students	B2 female students	B1 male students	B2 female students
C1 (Rural area)	ΣX=1131 MX=18.85 N=60	ΣX=1094 MX=18.23 N=60	ΣX=1196 MX=19.93 N=60	ΣX=1157 MX=19.28 N=60	ΣX=1206 MX=20.10 N=60	ΣX=1175 MX=19.58 N=60
C2 (Urban area)	ΣX=1175 MX=19.58 N=60	ΣX=1162 MX=19.37 N=60	ΣX=1186 MX=19.77 N=60	ΣX=1140 MX=19.00 N=60	ΣX=1074 MX=17.09 N=60	ΣX=1082 MX=18.03 N=60

The table no.**4.8.1** shows the mean score for Independent variables on Group oriented attitudes a part of mental health. The highest mean score was **20.10** of rural male Science students and the lowest mean score was **17.09** of urban male from Science faculty students.

Table 4.8.2
F calculation for Group oriented attitudes a part of mental health
(3x2x2 factorial designed)

Sources of variance	Sum of square	d.f.	Mean square	F	Significance level
Ass (Types of faculty)	49.83	2	24.91	2.46	N.S.
Bss (Sex)	44.29	1	44.29	4.37	0.05
Css (Area)	27.48	1	27.48	2.71	N S.
ABss	04.51	2	02.25	0.22	N S.
ACss	228.18	2	114.09	11.26	0.01
BCss	06.47	1	06.47	0.64	N S.
ABCss	07.18	2	03.60	0.36	N.S.
Wss	7173.07	708	10.13	-	-
Tss	7542.66	719	-	-	-

Significance levels df_1 0.05 = 3.85, 0.01= 6.66
df_2 0.05 = 3.00, 0.01= 4.63

The table no.**4.8.2** point out that F value of types of faculty variable was **2.46**, which was not significance at **0.05** levels. The F value of sex variables was 4.37, which was significance at **0.05** levels. The F value of Area variables was **2.71**, which was not significance at **0.05** levels. The F value of Interaction to types of faculty and Sex variables was **0.22**, which was not significance at **0.05** levels. The F value of Interaction to types of faculty and Area variables was **11.26**, which was significance at **0.01** levels.

The F value of Interaction to Sex and Area variables was **0.64**, which was not significance at **0.05** levels. The F value of Interaction to types of faculty, Sex and Area variables was **0.36**.

Ho_{36}: There is no significance difference of Group oriented attitudes a part of mental health based on types of faculty variable

Table No. 4.8.3
The mean score and F value for Types of faculty variable on Group oriented attitudes a part of mental health

No.	Variables	N	Mean	F	Significance
1	Arts faculty students (A_1)	240	19.01	**2.46**	**N.S.**
2	Commerce faculty students(A_2)	240	19.50		
3	Science faculty students(A3)	240	18.90		

Sig. levels df_2 = 0.05=3.00 / 0.01=4.63

Table No. 4.8.4
L.S.D. values for Types of faculty variable on Group oriented attitudes a part of mental health

Sr. No.	Pairs	Mean Diff.	Significance
1	A_1 vs. A_2	0.40	0.01
2	A_1 vs. A_3	0.11	N.S.
3	A_2 vs. A_3	0.60	0.01

Sig. levels for L.S.D. 0.05=0.17/ 0.01=0.22

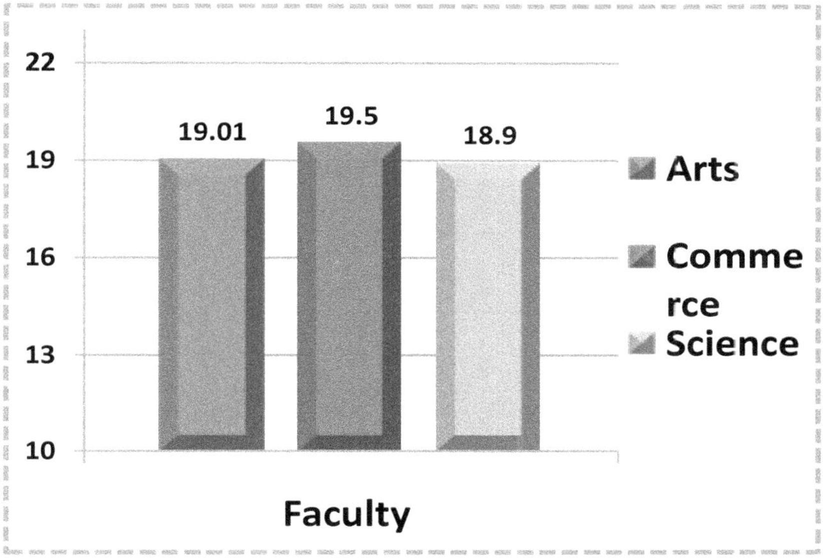

Figure No.36

Bar Chart of mean score of types of Faculty on Group oriented attitudes a part of mental health

It is clear from the table no.**4.8.3** the mean score for the Arts faculty respondents were **19.01**, the mean score of Commerce faculty respondents were **19.50** and the mean score of Science faculty respondents were **18.90**. The F value for types of Faculty variable was **2.46** which was not significant at 0.05 levels. Thus, our Ho_{36} was not rejected at 0.05 levels. So it can say that there was no significant difference between types of Faculty on Group oriented attitudes a part of mental health.

It could be seen from the table No.**4.8.4** and figure no.**36** L.S.D. values for types of faculty on Group oriented attitudes a part of mental health. The mean difference between Arts and Commerce faculty respondent was 0.40 which were not significant at 0.01 levels. The mean difference between Arts and Science faculty respondent was 0.11, which was not significant at 0.05 levels. The mean difference between Commerce and Science respondents was 0.60, which was significant difference at 0.01 levels.

Ho_{37}: There is no significance difference of Group oriented attitudes a part of mental health based on Sex variables.

Table No 4.8.5
Mean score of Sex variables on Group oriented attitudes a part of mental health

<table>
<tr><th>Variables</th><th>N</th><th>Mean score</th><th>F</th><th>Sig.</th></tr>
<tr><td>B_1 (Male)</td><td>360</td><td>19.39</td><td rowspan="2">4.37</td><td rowspan="2">0.05</td></tr>
<tr><td>B_2 (Female)</td><td>360</td><td>18.88</td></tr>
</table>

Significance levels df_2 =0.05=3.85/ 0.01=6.66

Table No. 4.8.6
L.S.D. values for Sex variable on Group oriented attitudes a part of mental health

<table>
<tr><th>No.</th><th>Variables(Sex)</th><th>N</th><th>Mean diff.</th><th>Significance</th></tr>
<tr><td>1</td><td>B_1 (Male)</td><td>360</td><td rowspan="2">0.51</td><td rowspan="2">0.05</td></tr>
<tr><td>2</td><td>B_2 (Female)</td><td>360</td></tr>
</table>

Significance levels for L.S.D. =0.05=0.47 / 0.01=0.61

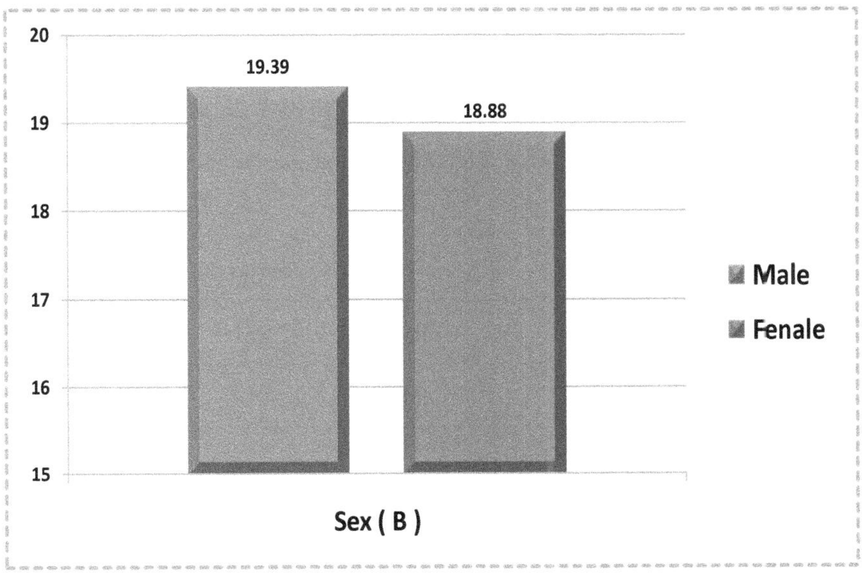

Figure No.37
Bar chart of mean score of sex variables on Group oriented attitudes a part of mental health

The table No. **4.8.5** indicated that the mean for male students was **19.39** and the mean for Female students was **18.88**. The F value for sex variables was **4.37,** which was significance at **0.05** levels. Hence, the **Ho**$_{37}$ was rejected and it could be said that there was significant mean difference between types of sex & their Group oriented attitudes a part of mental health score. So it saw the result and said that the male students are more Group oriented attitude a part of mental health than female students. Hence it concluded that Group oriented attitude a part of mental health was very affected factor for male students.

It is clear from the table No. **4.8.6** and figure **No.37** the L.S.D. for Types of Sex variables on Group oriented attitudes a part of mental health that the mean different between Male and Female students on Group oriented attitudes a part of mental health was **0.51**, which was Significance at **0.05** levels. Thus it concluded that the Male students are more Group oriented attitudes type Mentally Healthy than Female students. Hence it concluded that Group oriented attitudes a part of mental health was very affected factor for Male students.

Ho_{38}: There is no significance difference of Group oriented attitudes a part of mental health on Area variables.

Table No 4.8.7
Mean score and F value of Area variables on Group oriented attitudes a part of mental health

Variables	N	Mean score	F	Sig.
C_1 (Rural)	360	19.33	**2.71**	**N.S.**
C_2 (Urban)	360	18.94		

Significance levels df_2 =0.05=3.85 / 0.01=6.66

Table No. 4.8.8
L.S.D. values for Area variable on Group oriented attitudes a part of mental health

No.	Variables(Area)	N	Mean diff.	Significance
1	Rural students (c_1)	360	**0.39**	**N.S.**
2	Urban students (c_2)	360		

Significance levels for L.S.D. =0.05=0.47 / 0.01=0.61

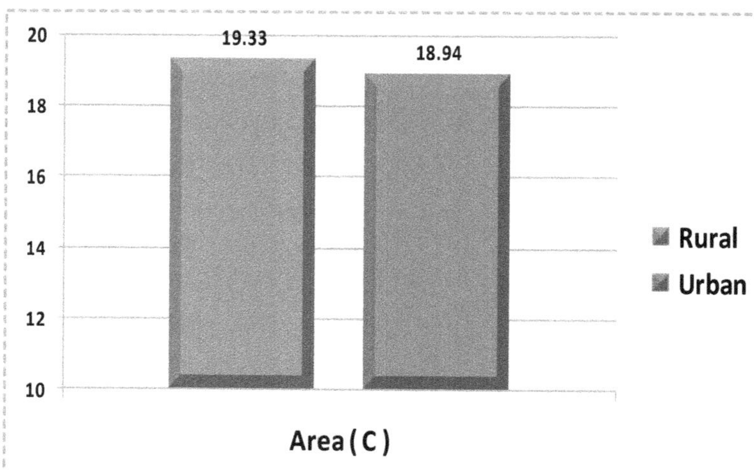

Figure No.38
Bar chart of mean score of Area variables of Group Oriented Attitudes a part of mental health

It could be seen from the table No. **4.8.7** that the mean for rural students was **19.33** and the mean for urban students was **18.94**. The F value for **Area** variables was **2.71,** which was not significance at **0.05** levels. Hence, the **Ho_{37}** was not rejected and it could be said that there was no significant mean difference between type of area & their Group Oriented Attitudes a part of mental health score.

It is observed from the table No. **4.8.8** and figure **No.38** the L.S.D. for types of Area variables on Group Oriented Attitudes a part of mental health that the mean different between Rural and Urban students on Group Oriented Attitudes a part of mental health was 0.39, which was not Significant at **0.05** levels. Thus it concluded that the rural students are more Group Oriented Attitudes type Mentally Healthy than Urban students. Hence it concluded that Group Oriented Attitudes a part of mental health was very affected factor for Male students.

Ho_{39}: There is no significance difference of Group Oriented Attitudes a part of mental health based on Interaction for type of faculty and Sex variables.

Table No 4.8.9

Interaction F for types of faculty and Sex variables on Group Oriented Attitudes a part of mental health

Variables	A_1 (Arts students)	A_2(commerce students)	A_3 (Science students)	F	Sig.
B_1 (Male students)	**19.22**	**19.85**	**19.00**	**0.22**	**N.S.**
B_2 (Female students)	**18.80**	**19.41**	**18.80**		

Significance levels df2 =0.05=3.00 / 0.01=4.63

Table No 4.8.10

A L.S.D. Table for Interaction of Types of faculty and Sex variables on Group Oriented Attitudes a part of mental health

Sr.NO.	Pairs	Mean Diff.	Significance
1	A_1B_1 vs. A_1B_2	0.42	N.S
2	A_1B_1 vs. A_2B_1	0.63	N.S.
3	A_1B_1 vs. A_2B_2	0.19	N.S

4	A_1B_1 vs. A_3B_1	0.22	N.S.
5	A_1B_1 vs. A_3B_2	0.42	N.S.
6	A_1B_2 vs. A_2B_1	1.05	0.01
7	A_1B_2 vs. A_2B_2	0.61	N.S.
8	A_1B_2 vs. A_3B_1	0.20	N.S.
9	A_1B_2 vs. A_3B_2	0.00	N.S.
10	A_2B_1 vs. A_2B_2	0.44	N.S.
11	A_2B_1 vs. A_3B_1	0.85	0.05
12	A_2B_1 vs. A_3B_2	1.05	0.01
13	A_2B_2 vs. A_3B_1	0.41	N.S.
14	A_2B_2 vs. A_3B_2	0.61	N.S.
15	A_3B_1 vs. A_3B_2	0.2	N.S.

Sig. levels for L.S.D. 0.05=0.80 / 0.01=1.05

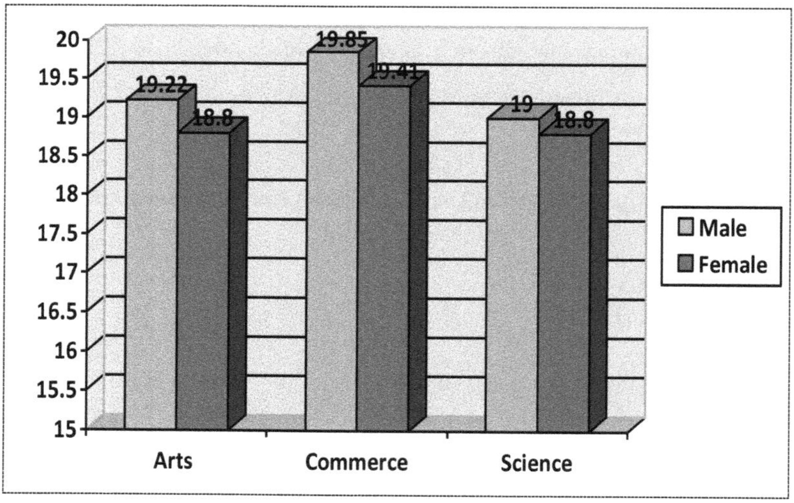

Figure No.39
Bar chart of mean score of Interaction of Types of faculty and Sex variables on Group Oriented Attitudes a part of mental health

It was indicated from the table No.**4.8.9** that the Interaction F for Type of faculty and Sex variables on Group Oriented Attitudes a part of mental health. The F value was **0.22**, which was not significance at **0.05** levels. Hence, the **Ho_{39}** was not rejected and it could be said that there was not significant mean difference between Types of faculty and sex variables & their Group Oriented Attitudes a part of mental health score.

The table no.**4.8.10** and figure **No.38** point out that L.S.D. for interaction of types of faculty and sex variables on Group Oriented Attitudes a part of mental health. It sees the result and said that most of the pairs are not significance at 0.05 or 0.01 levels. It also said that the highest mean score 19.85 was Commerce male students. The highest mean difference between A_1B_2 vs. A_2B_1 (Arts female students Vs. Commerce male students) was **1.50**, so it also said that it was big difference. The lowest mean difference between A_1B_2 v.A_3B_1 (Arts female students Vs. Science male students) was **0.00** on Group Oriented Attitudes a part of mental health. Hence, it see all the result and concluded that either all variables (faculties and sex) are affected on Group Oriented Attitudes a part of mental health or Group Oriented Attitudes a part of mental health was affected them.

Ho40: There is no significance difference of Group Oriented Attitudes a part of mental health based on Interaction for types of faculty and Area variables.

Table No 4.8.11

Interaction F for types of faculty and Area variables on Group Oriented Attitudes a part of mental health

Variables	A_1 (Arts students)	A_2 Commerce students	A_3 (Science students)	F	Sig.
C_1 (Rural)	**18.54**	**19.61**	**19.84**	**11.26**	**0.01**
C_2 (Urban)	**19.48**	**19.38**	**17.98**		

Significance levels df2 =0.05=3.00 / 0.01=4.63

Table No 4.8.12

A L.S.D. Table for Interaction of Types of faculty and Area variables on Group Oriented Attitudes a part of mental health

Sr.N0.	Pairs	Mean Diff.	Significance
1	A_1C_1 vs. A_1C_2	0.94	0.05
2	A_1C_1 vs. A_2C_1	1.07	0.01
3	A_1C_1 vs. A_2C_2	0.84	0.05
4	A_1C_1 vs.A_3C_1	1.30	0.01
5	A_1C_1 vs.A_3C_2	0.56	N.S.
6	A_1C_2 vs. A_2C_1	0.13	N.S.
7	A_1C_2 vs. A_2C_2	0.10	N.S.
8	A_1C_2 vs. A_3C_1	0.36	N.S.
9	A_1C_2 vs.A_3C_2	1.50	0.01
10	A_2C_1 vs.A_2C_2	0.23	N.S.
11	A_2C_1 vs.A_3C_1	0.23	N.S.
12	A_2C_1 vs.A_3C_2	1.63	0.01
13	A_2C_2 vs.A_3C_1	0.46	N.S.
14	A_2C_2 vs.A_3C_2	1.40	0.01
15	A_3C_1 vs.A_3C_2	1.86	0.01

Sig. levels for L.S.D. 0.05=0.80 / 0.01=1.05

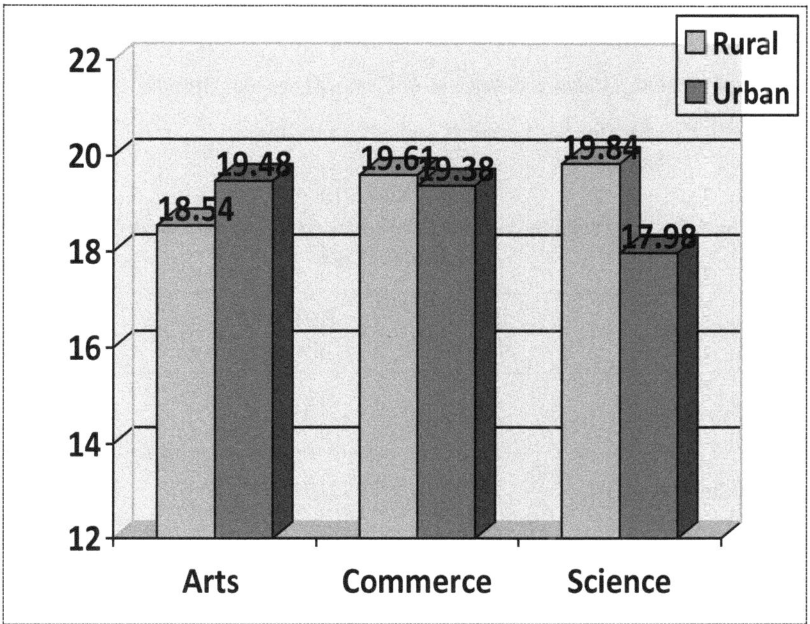

Figure No.40
Bar chart of interaction of Faculty and Area variables on Group Oriented Attitudes a part of mental health

It could be seen from the table No.**4.8.11** that the Interaction F for types of faculty and Area variables on Group Oriented Attitudes a part of mental health. The F value was **11.26**, which was significance at **0.01** levels. Hence, the **Ho$_{40}$** was rejected and it could be said that there was significant mean difference between types of faculty and area variables & their Group Oriented Attitudes a part of mental health score.

It is observed from the table no.**4.8.12** and figure**No.39** L.S.D. for interaction between the types of faculty and area variables on Group Oriented Attitudes a part of mental health. That it seen the result and said that the most of pairs significance at 0.05 or 0.01 levels. It also said the highest mean difference between A_2C_1vs.A_3C_2(Commerce rural students Vs. Science urban students) was **1.33**, so we can said that it was big difference. The lowest mean difference between A_1C_2vs.A_2C_1 (Arts urban students Vs. Commerce rural students) was **0.25** on Group Oriented Attitudes a part of mental health.

Ho_{41}: There is no significance difference of Group Oriented Attitudes a part of mental health based on for Sex variables and Area variables.

Table No 4.8.13

Interaction F for Sex variables and Area variables on Group Oriented Attitudes a part of mental health

Variables	B_1(Male students)	B_2 (Female students)	F	Sig.
Rural students (C_1)	19.63	19.03	**0.64**	**N.S.**
Urban students (C_2)	19.08	18.80		

Significance levels df_2 =0.05=3.85 / 0.01=6.66

Table No 4.8.14

A L.S.D. Table for Interaction of Sex and Area variables on Group Oriented Attitudes a part of mental health

Sr.NO.	Pairs	Mean Diff.	Significance
1	B_1C_1 vs. B_1C_2	0.55	N.S.
2	B_1C_1 vs. B_2C_1	0.60	N.S.
3	B_1C_1 vs. B_2C_2	0.83	N.S.
4	B_1C_2 vs.B_2C_1	0.05	N.S.
5	B_1C_2 vs. B_2C_2	0.28	N.S.
6	B_2C_1 vs. B_2C_2	0.23	N.S.

Sig. levels for L.S.D. 0.05=0.67 / 0.01=0.87

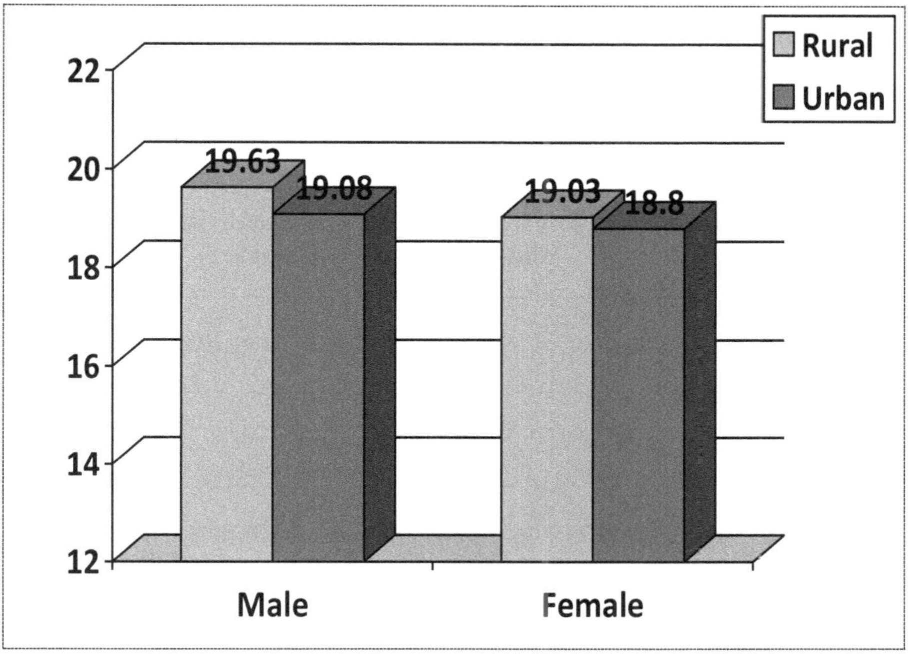

Figure No. 41

Bar chart of interaction of Sex and Area variables on Group Oriented Attitudes a part of mental health

The table No.**4.8.13** indicated that the Interaction F for Sex variables and Area variables on Group Oriented Attitudes a part of mental health. F value was **0.64**, which was not significance at **0.05** levels. Hence, the **Ho$_{41}$** was not rejected at 0.05 levels and it could be said that there was no significant mean difference between Sex variables and Area variables & their Group Oriented Attitudes a part of mental health score.

It is observed from the table **4.8.14** and figure No.**40** L.S.D. for interaction between the Sex variables and Area variables on Group Oriented Attitudes a part of mental health, that it seen the result and said that most of pairs are not significance at 0.05 levels.

Ho_{42}: There is no significance difference of Group Oriented Attitudes a part of mental health based on Interaction for types of faculty, Sex and Area variables.

Table No 4.8.15
Interaction F for types of Faculty, Sex and Area variables on Group Oriented Attitudes a part of mental health

variables	A_1(Arts students)		A_2(Commerce students)		A_3(Science students)		F	Sig.
	B_1 male students	B_2 female students	B_1 male students	B_2 female students	B_1 male students	B_2 female students		
C_1	18.85	18.23	19.93	19.28	20.10	19.58	0.36	N.S.
C_2	19.58	19.37	19.77	19.00	17.90	18.03		

Significance levels df_1 =0.05=3.00 / 0.01=4.63

Table No 4.8.16
A L.S.D. Table for Interaction of types of faculty, Sex and Area variables on Group Oriented Attitudes a part of mental health

Sr.N0.	Pairs	Mean Diff.	Significance
1	$A_1B_1C_1$ vs. $A_1B_1C_2$	0.73	N.S.
2	$A_1B_1C_1$ vs. $A_1B_2C_1$	0.62	N.S.
3	$A_1B_1C_1$ vs. $A_1B_2C_2$	0.52	N.S.
4	$A_1B_1C_1$ vs. $A_2B_1C_1$	1.08	0.05
5	$A_1B_1C_1$ vs. $A_2B_1C_2$	0.92	N.S.
6	$A_1B_1C_1$ vs. $A_2B_2C_1$	0.43	N.S.
7	$A_1B_1C_1$ vs. $A_2B_2C_2$	0.15	N.S.
8	$A_1B_1C_1$ vs. $A_3B_1C_1$	1.25	0.05
9	$A_1B_1C_1$ vs. $A_3B_1C_2$	0.95	N.S.
10	$A_1B_1C_1$ vs. $A_3B_2C_1$	0.73	N.S.
11	$A_1B_1C_1$ vs. $A_3B_2C_2$	0.82	N.S.
12	$A_1B_1C_2$ vs. $A_1B_2C_1$	1.35	0.05

13	$A_1B_1C_2$ vs. $A_1B_2C_2$	0.21	N.S.
14	$A_1B_1C_2$ vs. $A_2B_1C_1$	0.35	N.S.
15	$A_1B_1C_2$ vs. $A_2B_1C_2$	0.19	N.S.
16	$A_1B_1C_2$ vs. $A_2B_2C_1$	0.30	N.S.
17	$A_1B_1C_2$ vs. $A_2B_2C_2$	0.58	N.S.
18	$A_1B_1C_2$ vs. $A_3B_1C_1$	0.52	N.S.
19	$A_1B_1C_2$ vs. $A_3B_1C_2$	1.68	0.01
20	$A_1B_1C_2$ vs. $A_3B_2C_1$	0.00	N.S.
21	$A_1B_1C_2$ vs. $A_3B_2C_2$	1.55	0.01
22	$A_1B_2C_1$ vs. $A_1B_2C_2$	1.14	0.05
23	$A_1B_2C_1$ vs. $A_2B_1C_1$	1.70	0.01
24	$A_1B_2C_1$ vs. $A_2B_1C_2$	1.54	0.01
25	$A_1B_2C_1$ vs. $A_2B_2C_1$	1.05	0.05
26	$A_1B_2C_1$ vs. $A_2B_2C_2$	0.77	N.S.
27	$A_1B_2C_1$ vs. $A_3B_1C_1$	1.87	0.01
28	$A_1B_2C_1$ vs. $A_3B_1C_2$	0.33	N.S.
29	$A_1B_2C_1$ vs. $A_3B_2C_1$	1.35	0.05
30	$A_1B_2C_1$ vs. $A_3B_2C_2$	0.20	N.S.
31	$A_1B_2C_2$ vs. $A_2B_1C_1$	0.56	N.S.
32	$A_1B_2C_2$ vs. $A_2B_1C_2$	0.40	N.S.
33	$A_1B_2C_2$ vs. $A_2B_2C_1$	0.09	N.S.
34	$A_1B_2C_2$ vs. $A_2B_2C_2$	0.37	N.S.
35	$A_1B_2C_2$ vs. $A_3B_1C_1$	0.73	N.S.
36	$A_1B_2C_2$ vs. $A_3B_1C_2$	1.47	0.05
37	$A_1B_2C_2$ vs. $A_3B_2C_1$	0.21	N.S.
38	$A_1B_2C_2$ vs. $A_3B_2C_2$	1.34	0.05
39	$A_2B_1C_1$ vs. $A_2B_1C_2$	0.16	N.S.
40	$A_2B_1C_1$ vs. $A_2B_2C_1$	0.65	N.S.
41	$A_2B_1C_1$ vs. $A_2B_2C_2$	0.93	N.S.
42	$A_2B_1C_1$ vs. $A_3B_1C_1$	0.17	N.S.
43	$A_2B_1C_1$ vs. $A_3B_1C_2$	2.03	0.01
44	$A_2B_1C_1$ vs. $A_3B_2C_1$	0.35	N.S.
45	$A_2B_1C_1$ vs. $A_3B_2C_2$	1.90	0.01

46	$A_2B_1C_2$ vs. $A_2B_2C_1$	0.49	N.S.
47	$A_2B_1C_2$ vs. $A_2B_2C_2$	0.77	N.S.
48	$A_2B_1C_2$ vs. $A_3B_1C_1$	0.33	N.S.
49	$A_2B_1C_2$ vs. $A_3B_1C_2$	1.87	0.01
50	$A_2B_1C_2$ vs. $A_3B_2C_1$	0.19	N.S.
51	$A_2B_1C_2$ vs. $A_3B_2C_2$	1.74	0.01
52	$A_2B_2C_1$ vs. $A_2B_2C_2$	0.28	N.S.
53	$A_2B_2C_1$ vs. $A_3B_1C_1$	0.82	N.S.
54	$A_2B_2C_1$ vs. $A_3B_1C_2$	1.38	0.05
55	$A_2B_2C_1$ vs. $A_3B_2C_1$	0.30	N.S.
56	$A_2B_2C_1$ vs. $A_3B_2C_2$	1.25	0.05
57	$A_2B_2C_2$ vs. $A_3B_1C_1$	1.10	0.05
58	$A_2B_2C_2$ vs. $A_3B_1C_2$	1.10	0.05
59	$A_2B_2C_2$ vs. $A_3B_2C_1$	0.58	N.S.
60	$A_2B_2C_2$ vs. $A_3B_2C_2$	0.97	N.S.
61	$A_3B_1C_1$ vs. $A_3B_1C_2$	2.20	0.01
62	$A_3B_1C_1$ vs. $A_3B_2C_1$	0.52	N.S.
63	$A_3B_1C_1$ vs. $A_3B_2C_2$	2.07	0.01
64	$A_3B_1C_2$ vs. $A_3B_2C_1$	1.68	0.01
65	$A_3B_1C_2$vs. $A_3B_2C_2$	0.13	N.S.
66	$A_3B_2.C_1$ vs. $A_3B_2C_2$	1.55	0.01

Sig. levels for L.S.D. 0.05=1.01/ 0.01=1.49

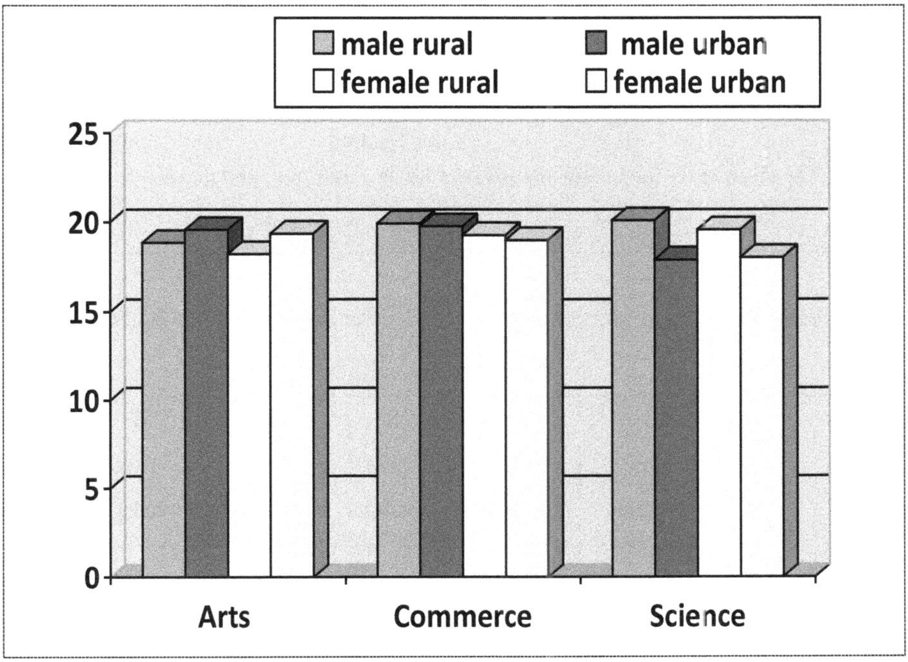

Figure No.42
The bar chart of interaction between the types of faculty, sex and area variables on Group oriented attitudes a part of mental health

It is observed from the table No.**4.8.15** that the Interaction F for types of Faculty, Sex variables and Area variables on Group Oriented Attitudes a part of mental health. F value was **0.36**, which was not significance at **0.05** levels. Hence, the **Ho_{42}** was not rejected at 0.05 levels and it could be said that there was no significant mean difference between Sex variables and Area variables & their Group Oriented Attitudes a part of mental health score.

It could be seen from the table **4.8.16** the **L.S.D.** for interaction between the Types of faculty, Sex variables and Area variables on Group Oriented Attitudes a part of mental health, that we seen the result and said that most of pairs are significance at 0.05 levels. It also said highest mean difference between B_1C_1vs. B_2C_2 (male rural students vs. female urban students) was 1.95, so we said that it was big difference. The lowest mean difference score between B_2C_1 vs. B_2C_2 (female rural students vs. female urban students) was 0.10 on Group oriented Attitude a part of mental health.

4.9.1 The Respondents socio personal variables and their 3x2x2 factorial design for Environmental mastery a part of mental health

Table No.4.9.1
The mean score for Independent variables on Environmental mastery a part of mental health

Variables	A1(Arts faculty)		A2(Commerce faculty)		A3(Science faculty)	
	B1 male students	B2 female students	B1 male students	B2 female students	B1 male students	B2 female students
C1 (Rural area)	∑X=1077 MX=17.95 N=60	∑X=1078 MX=17.97 N=60	∑X=1153 MX=19.22 N=60	∑X=1086 MX=18.10 N=60	∑X=1167 MX=19.45 N=60	∑X=1132 MX=18.87 N=60
C2 (Urban area)	∑X=1086 MX=18.10 N=60	∑X=1101 MX=18.3 N=60	∑X=1171 MX=19.52 N=60	∑X=1050 MX=17.50 N=60	∑X=1036 MX=17.27 N=60	∑X=1079 MX=17.98 N=60

The table no.**4.9.1** shows the mean score for Independent variables on Group oriented attitudes a part of mental health. The highest mean score was **19.45** of rural male Science students and the lowest mean score was **17.50** of urban male from commerce faculty students.

Table 4.9.2

F calculation for Environmental mastery a part of Mental health (3x2x2 factorial designed)

Sources of variance	Sum of square	d.f.	Mean square	F	Significance level
Ass (Types of faculty)	29.48	2	14.74	1.70	N.S.
Bss (Sex)	42.39	1	42.39	4.88	0.05
Css (Area)	37.61	1	37.61	4.33	0.05
ABss	107.10	2	53.55	6.17	0.01
ACss	111.09	2	55.55	6.40	0.01
BCss	02.10	1	02.10	0.24	N.S.
ABCss	37.05	2	18.53	2.14	N.S.
Wss	6144.50	708	8.68	-	-
Tss	6512.98	719	-	-	-

Significance levels df_1 0.05 = 3.85, 0.01= 6.66
df_2 0.05 = 3.00, 0.01= 4.63

The table no.**4.9.2** point out that F value of types of faculty variable was **1.70**, which was not significance at **0.05** levels. The F value of sex variables was **4.88**, which was significance at **0.05** levels. The F value of Area variables was **4.33**, which was significance at **0.05** levels. The F value of Interaction to types of faculty and Sex variables was **6.17**, which was significance at **0.01** levels. The F value of Interaction to types of faculty and Area variables was **6.40**, which was significance at **0.01** levels.

The F value of Interaction to Sex and Area variables was **0.24**, which was not significance at **0.05** levels. The F value of Interaction to types of faculty, Sex and Area variables was **2.14**.

Ho_{43}: There is no significance difference of Environmental mastery a part of mental health based on types of faculty variable.

Table No. 4.9.3

The mean score and F value for Types of faculty variable on Environmental mastery a part of mental health

No.	Variables	N	Mean	F	Significance
1	Arts faculty students (A_1)	240	18.10	**1.70**	**N.S.**
2	Commerce faculty students(A_2)	240	18.51		
3	Science faculty students(A3)	240	18.39		

Significance levels df_2 = 0.05=3.00 / 0.01=4.63

Table No. 4.9.4

L.S.D. values for Types of faculty variable on Environmental mastery a part of mental health

Sr.No.	Pairs	Mean Diff.	Significance
1	A_1 vs. A_2	0.48	N.S.
2	A_1 vs. A_3	0.29	N.S.
3	A_2 vs. A_3	0.60	0.01

Sig. levels for L.S.D. 0.05=1.04 / 0.01=1.36

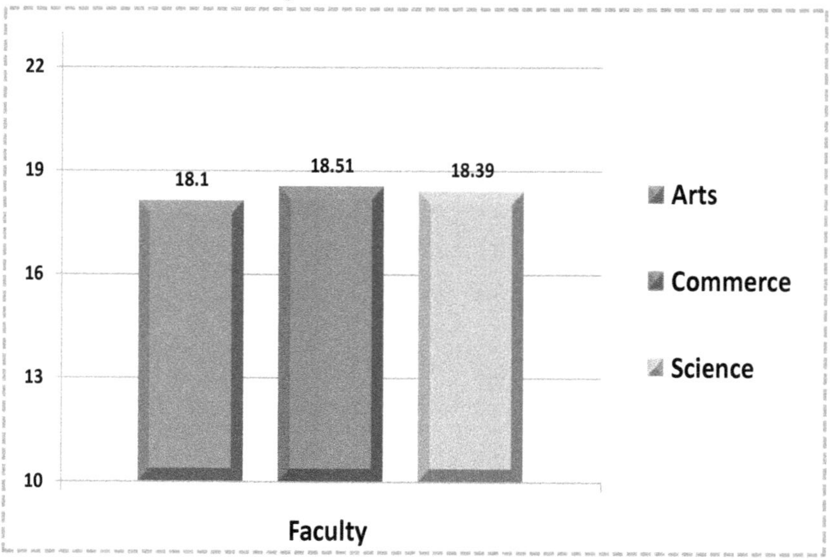

Figure No.43

Bar Chart of mean score of types of Faculty on Environmental mastery a part of mental health

It is clear from the table no.**4.9.3** the mean score for the Arts faculty respondents were **18.10**, the mean score of Commerce faculty respondents were **18.51** and the mean score of Science faculty respondents were **18.39**. The F value for types of Faculty variable was **1.70** which was not significant at 0.05 levels. Thus, our Ho_{43} was not rejected at 0.05 levels. So it can say that there was no significant difference between types of Faculty on Environmental mastery a part of mental health.

It could be seen from the table No.**4.9.4** and figure no.**43** L.S.D. values for types of faculty on Environmental mastery a part of mental health. The mean difference between Arts and Commerce faculty respondent was 0.48 which were not significant at 0.05 levels. The mean difference between Arts and Science faculty respondent was 0.29, which was not significant at 0.05 levels. The mean difference between Commerce and Science respondents was 0.19, which was significant difference at 0.01 levels.

Ho_{44}: There is no significance difference of Environmental mastery a part of mental health based on Sex variables.

Table No 4.9.5
Mean score of Sex variables on Environmental mastery a part of mental health

Variables	N	Mean score	F	Sig.
B_1 (Male)	360	18.61	**4.88**	**0.05**
B_2 (Female)	360	18.11		

Significance levels df_2 =0.05=3.85 / 0.01=6.66

Table No. 4.9.6
L.S.D. values for Sex variable on Environmental mastery a part of mental health

No.	Variables(Sex)	N	Mean diff.	Significance
1	B_1 (Male)	360	**0.50**	0.05
2	B_2 (Female)	360		

Significance levels for L.S.D. =0.05=0.43/ 0.01=0.56

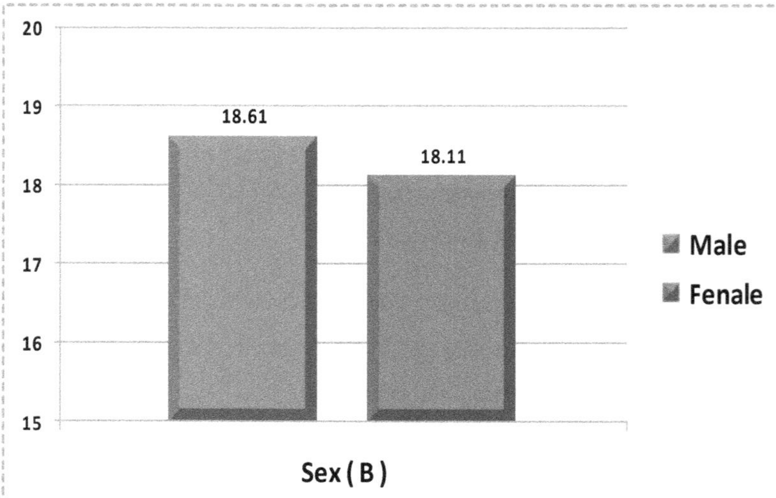

Figure No.44
Bar chart of mean score of sex variables on Environmental mastery a part of mental health

The table No. **4.8.5** indicated that the mean for male students was **118.61** and the mean for Female students was **18.11**. The F value for sex variables was **4.88,** which was significance at **0.05** levels. Hence, the **Ho$_{44}$** was rejected and it could be said that there was significant mean difference between types of sex & their Environmental mastery a part of mental health score. So it saw the result and said that the male students are more Environmental mastery a part of mental health than female students. Hence it concluded that a part of mental health was very affected factor for male students.

It is clear from the table No. **4.9.6** and figure **No.44** the L.S.D. for Types of Sex variables on Environmental mastery a part of mental health that the mean different between Male and Female students on Environmental mastery a part of mental health was **0.50**, which was Significance at **0.05** levels. Thus it concluded that the Male students are more Environmental mastery type Mentally Healthy than Female students. Hence it concluded that Environmental mastery a part of mental health was very affected factor for Male students.

Ho_{45}: There is no significance difference of Environmental mastery a part of mental health on Area variables.

Table No 4.9.7
Mean score and F value of Area variables on Environmental mastery a part of mental health

Variables	N	Mean score	F	Sig.
C_1 (Rural)	360	18.58	**0.45**	**N.S.**
C_2 (Urban)	360	18.13		

Significance levels df_2 =0.05=3.85 / 0.01=6.66

Table No. 4.9.8
L.S.D. values for Area variable on Environmental mastery a part of mental health

No.	Variables(Area)	N	Mean diff.	Significance
1	Rural students (c_1)	360	**0.45**	**0.05**
2	Urban students (c_2)	360		

Significance levels for L.S.D. =0.05=0.43 / 0.01=0.56

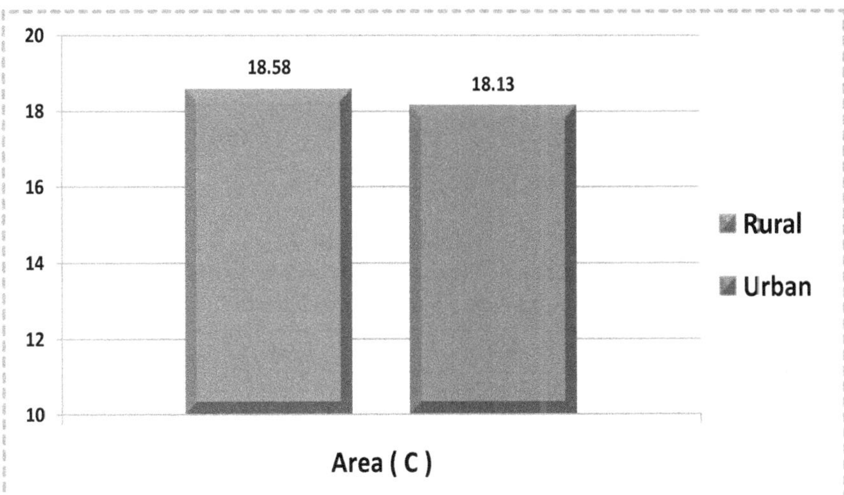

Figure No.45
Bar chart of mean score of Area variables of Environmental mastery a part of mental health

It could be seen from the table No. **4.9.7** that the mean for rural students was **18.58** and the mean for urban students was **18.13**. The F value for **Area** variables was **0.45,** which was significance at **0.05** levels. Hence, the **Ho_{45}** was not rejected and it could be said that there was no significant mean difference between type of area & their Environmental mastery a part of mental health score.

It is observed from the table No. **4.9.8** and figure **No.45** the L.S.D. for types of Area variables on Environmental mastery a part of mental health that the mean different between Rural and Urban students on Environmental mastery a part of mental health was 0.45, which was Significant at **0.05** levels. Thus it concluded that the rural students are more Environmental mastery type Mentally Healthy than Urban students. Hence it concluded that Environmental mastery a part of mental health was very affected factor for Male students.

Ho_{46}: There is no significance difference of Environmental mastery a part of mental health based on Interaction for type of faculty and Sex variables.

Table No 4.9.9
Interaction F for types of faculty and Sex variables on Environmental mastery a part of mental health

Variables	A_1 (Arts students)	A_2(commerce students)	A_3 (Science students)	F	Sig.
B_1 (Male students)	**18.03**	**19.37**	**18.35**	**6.17**	**0.01**
B_2 (Female students)	**18.16**	**17.80**	**18.43**		

Significance levels df2 =0.05=3.00 / 0.01=4.60

Table No 4.9.10
A L.S.D. Table for Interaction of Types of faculty and Sex variables on Environmental mastery a part of mental health

Sr.N0.	Pairs	Mean Diff.	Significance
1	A_1B_1 vs. A_1B_2	0.13	N.S
2	A_1B_1 vs. A_2B_1	1.34	0.01
3	A_1B_1 vs. A_2B_2	0.23	0.01
4	A_1B_1 vs.A_3B_1	0.32	0.01
5	A_1B_1 vs.A_3B_2	0.40	0.01

6	A_1B_2 vs. A_2B_1	1.21	0.01
7	A_1B_2 vs. A_2B_2	0.36	0.01
8	A_1B_2 vs. A_3B_1	0.19	0.05
9	A_1B_2 vs.A_3B_2	0.27	0.01
10	A_2B_1 vs.A_2B_2	1.57	0.01
11	A_2B_1 vs.A_3B_1	1.02	0.01
12	A_2B_1 vs.A_3B_2	2.94	0.01
13	A_2B_2 vs.A_3B_1	0.55	0.01
14	A_2B_2 vs.A_3B_2	0.63	0.01
15	A_3B_1 vs.A_3B_2	0.08	N.S.

Sig. levels for L.S.D. 0.05=0.16 / 0.01=0.21

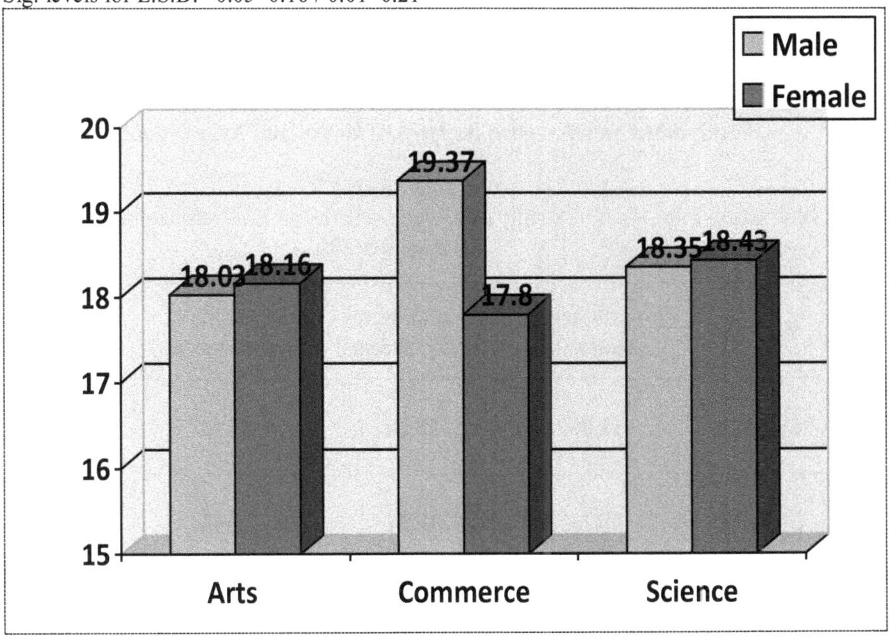

Figure No.46
Bar chart of mean score of Interaction of Types of faculty and Sex variables on Environmental mastery a part of mental health

It was indicated from the table No.**4.9.9** that the Interaction F for Type of faculty and Sex variables on Environmental mastery a part of mental health. The F value was **6.17**, which was significance at **0.01** levels. Hence, the **Ho_{46}** was rejected and it could be said that there was significant mean difference between Types of faculty and sex variables & their Environmental mastery a part of mental health score.

The table no.**4.9.10** and figure **No.46** point out that L.S.D. for interaction of types of faculty and sex variables on Environmental mastery a part of mental health. It sees the result and said that most of the pairs are not significance at 0.05 or 0.01 levels. The highest mean difference between A_1B_2 vs. A_2B_1 (Arts female students Vs. Commerce male students) was **1.50**, so it also said that it was big difference. The lowest mean difference between A_1B_2 vsA_3B_1 (Arts female students Vs. Science male students) was **0.00** on Environmental mastery a part of mental health. Hence, it sees all the result and concluded that either all variables (faculties and sex) are affected on Environmental mastery a part of mental health or Environmental mastery a part of mental health was affected them.

Ho_{47}: There is no significance difference of Environmental mastery a part of mental health based on interaction for types of faculty and Area variables.

Table No 4.9.11
Interaction F for types of faculty and Area variables on Environmental mastery a part of mental health

Variables	A_1(Arts faculty students)	A_2 (Commerce faculty students)	A_3(Science faculty students)	F	Sig.
C_1 (Rural)	**17.96**	**18.66**	**19.16**	**6.40**	**0.01**
C_2 (Urban)	**18.23**	**18.51**	**17.63**		

Significance levels df2 =0.05=3.00 / 0.01=4.63

Table No 4.9.12
A L.S.D. Table for Interaction of Types of faculty and Area variables on Environmental mastery a part of mental health

Sr.N0.	Pairs	Mean Diff.	Significance
1	A_1C_1 vs. A_1C_2	0.27	0.01
2	A_1C_1 vs. A_2C_1	0.70	0.01
3	A_1C_1 vs. A_2C_2	0.55	0.01
4	A_1C_1 vs.A_3C_1	1.20	0.01

5	A_1C_1 vs. A_3C_2	0.33	0.01
6	A_1C_2 vs. A_2C_1	0.43	0.01
7	A_1C_2 vs. A_2C_2	0.28	0.01
8	A_1C_2 vs. A_3C_1	0.93	0.01
9	A_1C_2 vs. A_3C_2	0.60	0.01
10	A_2C_1 vs. A_2C_2	0.15	N.S.
11	A_2C_1 vs. A_3C_1	0.50	0.01
12	A_2C_1 vs. A_3C_2	1.03	0.01
13	A_2C_2 vs. A_3C_1	0.65	0.01
14	A_2C_2 vs. A_3C_2	0.88	0.01
15	A_3C_1 vs. A_3C_2	1.53	0.01

Sig. levels for L.S.D. 0.05=0.16 / 0.01=0.21

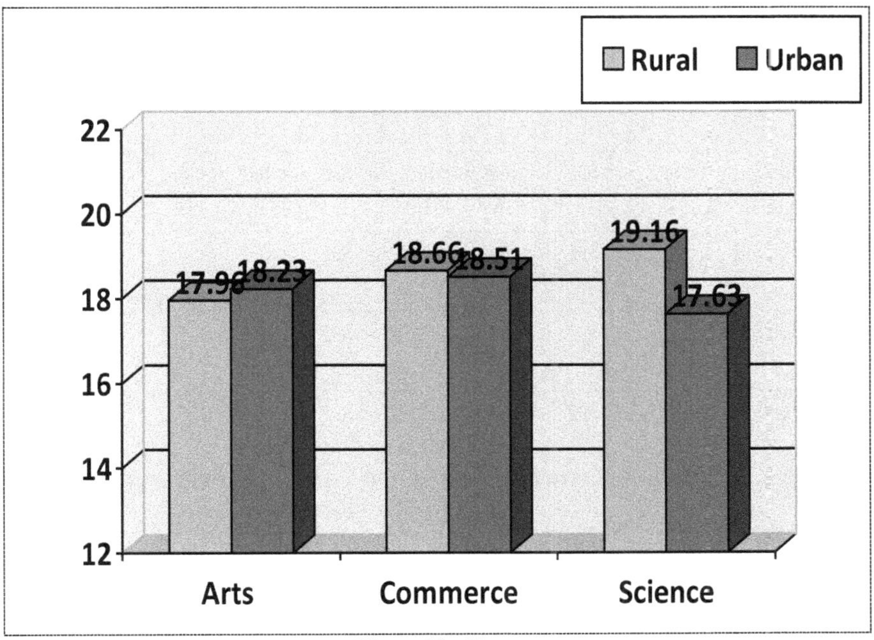

Figure No.47

Bar chart of interaction of Faculty and Area variables on Environmental mastery a part of mental health

It could be seen from the table No.**4.9.11** that the Interaction F for types of faculty and Area variables on Environmental mastery a part of mental health. The F value was **0.24**, which was not significance at **0.05** levels. Hence, the **Ho_{47}** was not rejected and it could be said that there was significant mean difference between types of faculty and area variables & their Environmental mastery a part of mental health score.

It is observed from the table no.**4.9.12** and figure**No.47** L.S.D. for interaction between the types of faculty and area variables on Environmental mastery a part of mental health. That it seen the result and said that the most of pairs significance at 0.05 or 0.01 levels. It also said the highest mean difference between A_2C_1 vs.A_3C_2 (Science rural students Vs. Science urban students) was **1.53**, so it can said that it was big difference. The lowest mean difference between A_1C_2vs.A_2C_1 (Commerce rural students Vs. Commerce urban students) was **0.15** on Environmental mastery a part of mental health.

Ho_{48}: There is no significance difference of Environmental mastery a part of mental health based on for Sex variables and Area variables.

Table No 4.9.13
Interaction F for Sex variables and Area variables on Environmental mastery a part of mental health

Variables	B_1(Male students)	B_2 (Female students)	F	Sig.
Rural students (C_1)	18.87	18.31	**0.24**	**N.S.**
Urban students (C_2)	19.29	17.94		

Significance levels df_2 =0.05=3.85 / 0.01=6.66

Table No 4.9.14
A L.S.D. Table for Interaction of Sex and Area variables on Environmental mastery a part of mental health

Sr.No.	Pairs	Mean Diff.	Significance
1	B_1C_1 vs. B_1C_2	0.42	N.S.
2	B_1C_1 vs. B_2C_1	0.56	N.S.
3	B_1C_1 vs. B_2C_2	0.93	0.01
4	B_1C_2 vs.B_2C_1	0.98	0.01
5	B_1C_2 vs. B_2C_2	1.35	0.01
6	B_2C_1 vs. B_2C_2	0.37	0.01

Sig. levels for L.S.D. 0.05=0.61/0.01=0.79

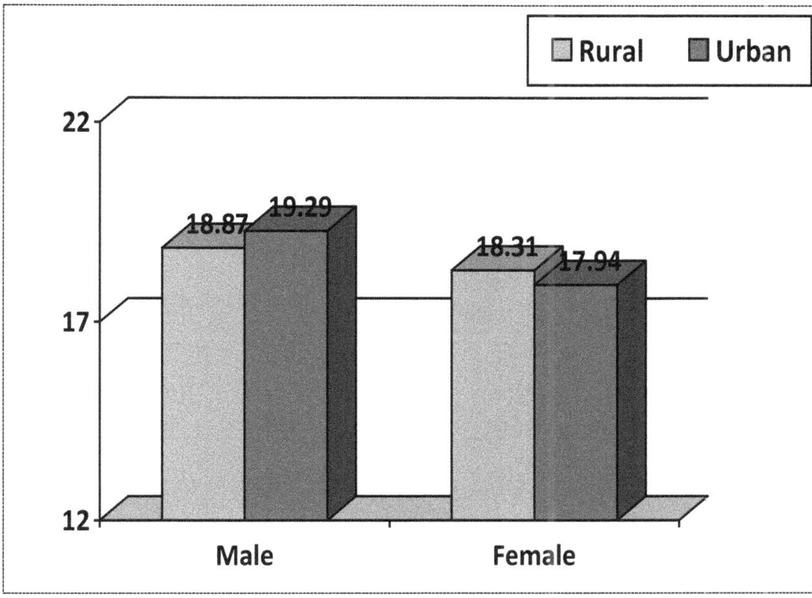

Figure No. 48
Bar chart of interaction of Sex and Area variables on Environmental mastery a part of mental health

The table No.**4.9.13** indicated that the Interaction F for Sex variables and Area variables on Group Oriented Attitudes a part of mental health. F value was **0.24**, which was not significance at **0.05** levels. Hence, the **Ho$_{48}$** was not rejected at 0.05 levels and it could be said that there was no significant mean difference between Sex variables and Area variables & their Environmental mastery a part of mental health score.

It is observed from the table **4.9.14** and figure No.**48** L.S.D. for interaction between the Sex variables and Area variables on Environmental mastery a part of mental health, that it seen the result and said that most of pairs are not significance at 0.05 levels.

H_{049}: There is no significance difference of Environmental mastery a part of mental health based on Interaction for types of faculty, Sex and Area variables.

Table No 4.9.15
Interaction F for types of Faculty, Sex and Area variables on Environmental mastery a part of mental health

Vari.	A_1(Arts students)		A_2(Commerce students)		A_3(Science students)		F	Sig.
	B_1 male students	B_2 female students	B_1 male students	B_2 female students	B_1 male students	B_2 female students		
C_1	17.95	17.97	19.22	18.10	19.45	18.87	2.14	N.S.
C_2	18.10	18.35	19.52	17.50	17.27	17.98		

Significance levels df_1 =0.05=3.00 / 0.01=4.63

Table No 4.9.16
A L.S.D. Table for Interaction of types of faculty, Sex and Area variables on Environmental mastery a part of mental health

Sr.NO.	Pairs	Mean Diff.	Significance
1	$A_1B_1C_1$ vs. $A_1B_1C_2$	0.15	N.S.
2	$A_1B_1C_1$ vs. $A_1B_2C_1$	0.02	N.S.
3	$A_1B_1C_1$ vs. $A_1B_2C_2$	0.40	N.S.
4	$A_1B_1C_1$ vs. $A_2B_1C_1$	1.27	0.05
5	$A_1B_1C_1$ vs. $A_2B_1C_2$	1.57	0.01
6	$A_1B_1C_1$ vs. $A_2B_2C_1$	0.15	N.S.
7	$A_1B_1C_1$ vs. $A_2B_2C_2$	0.45	N.S.
8	$A_1B_1C_1$ vs. $A_3B_1C_1$	1.50	0.01
9	$A_1B_1C_1$ vs. $A_3B_1C_2$	0.68	N.S.
10	$A_1B_1C_1$ vs. $A_3B_2C_1$	0.92	N.S.
11	$A_1B_1C_1$ vs. $A_3B_2C_2$	0.03	N.S.
12	$A_1B_1C_2$ vs. $A_1B_2C_1$	0.13	N.S.

13	$A_1B_1C_2$ vs. $A_1B_2C_2$	0.25	N.S.
14	$A_1B_1C_2$ vs. $A_2B_1C_1$	1.12	0.05
15	$A_1B_1C_2$ vs. $A_2B_1C_2$	1.42	0.01
16	$A_1B_1C_2$ vs. $A_2B_2C_1$	0.00	N.S.
17	$A_1B_1C_2$ vs. $A_2B_2C_2$	0.60	N.S.
18	$A_1B_1C_2$ vs. $A_3B_1C_1$	1.35	0.05
19	$A_1B_1C_2$ vs. $A_3B_1C_2$	0.68	N.S.
20	$A_1B_1C_2$ vs. $A_3B_2C_1$	0.77	N.S.
21	$A_1B_1C_2$ vs. $A_3B_2C_2$	0.12	N.S.
22	$A_1B_2C_1$ vs. $A_1B_2C_2$	0.38	N.S.
23	$A_1B_2C_1$ vs. $A_2B_1C_1$	1.25	0.05
24	$A_1B_2C_1$ vs. $A_2B_1C_2$	1.55	0.01
25	$A_1B_2C_1$ vs. $A_2B_2C_1$	0.13	N.S.
26	$A_1B_2C_1$ vs. $A_2B_2C_2$	0.47	N.S.
27	$A_1B_2C_1$ vs. $A_3B_1C_1$	1.48	0.01
28	$A_1B_2C_1$ vs. $A_3B_1C_2$	0.70	N.S.
29	$A_1B_2C_1$ vs. $A_3B_2C_1$	0.90	N.S.
30	$A_1B_2C_1$ vs. $A_3B_2C_2$	0.01	N.S.
31	$A_1B_2C_2$ vs. $A_2B_1C_1$	0.87	N.S.
32	$A_1B_2C_2$ vs. $A_2B_1C_2$	1.17	0.05
33	$A_1B_2C_2$ vs. $A_2B_2C_1$	0.25	N.S.
34	$A_1B_2C_2$ vs. $A_2B_2C_2$	0.85	N.S.
35	$A_1B_2C_2$ vs. $A_3B_1C_1$	1.10	0.05
36	$A_1B_2C_2$ vs. $A_3B_1C_2$	1.08	0.05
37	$A_1B_2C_2$ vs. $A_3B_2C_1$	0.52	N.S.
38	$A_1B_2C_2$ vs. $A_3B_2C_2$	0.37	N.S.
39	$A_2B_1C_1$ vs. $A_2B_1C_2$	0.30	N.S.
40	$A_2B_1C_1$ vs. $A_2B_2C_1$	1.12	0.05
41	$A_2B_1C_1$ vs. $A_2B_2C_2$	1.72	0.01
42	$A_2B_1C_1$ vs. $A_3B_1C_1$	0.23	N.S
43	$A_2B_1C_1$ vs. $A_3B_1C_2$	1.95	0.01
44	$A_2B_1C_1$ vs. $A_3B_2C_1$	0.35	N.S
45	$A_2B_1C_1$ vs. $A_3B_2C_2$	1.24	0.05

46	$A_2B_1C_2$ vs. $A_2B_2C_1$	1.42	0.01
47	$A_2B_1C_2$ vs. $A_2B_2C_2$	2.02	0.01
48	$A_2B_1C_2$ vs. $A_3B_1C_1$	0.07	N.S.
49	$A_2B_1C_2$ vs. $A_3B_1C_2$	2.25	0.01
50	$A_2B_1C_2$ vs. $A_3B_2C_1$	0.65	N.S.
51	$A_2B_1C_2$ vs. $A_3B_2C_2$	1.54	0.01
52	$A_2B_2C_1$ vs. $A_2B_2C_2$	0.60	N.S.
53	$A_2B_2C_1$ vs. $A_3B_1C_1$	1.35	0.05
54	$A_2B_2C_1$ vs. $A_3B_1C_2$	0.83	N.S.
55	$A_2B_2C_1$ vs. $A_3B_2C_1$	0.77	N.S.
56	$A_2B_2C_1$ vs. $A_3B_2C_2$	0.12	N.S.
57	$A_2B_2C_2$ vs. $A_3B_1C_1$	1.95	0.01
58	$A_2B_2C_2$ vs. $A_3B_1C_2$	0.23	N.S.
59	$A_2B_2C_2$ vs. $A_3B_2C_1$	1.37	0.05
60	$A_2B_2C_2$ vs. $A_3B_2C_2$	0.48	N.S.
61	$A_3B_1C_1$ vs. $A_3B_1C_2$	2.18	0.01
62	$A_3B_1C_1$ vs. $A_3B_2C_1$	0.58	N.S.
63	$A_3B_1C_1$ vs. $A_3B_2C_2$	1.47	0.01
64	$A_3B_1C_2$ vs. $A_3B_2C_1$	1.60	0.01
65	$A_3B_1C_2$vs. $A_3B_2C_2$	0.71	N.S.
66	$A_3B_{2.}C_1$ vs. $A_3B_2C_2$	0.89	N.S.

Sig. levels for L.S.D. 0.05=1.06 / 0.01=1.38

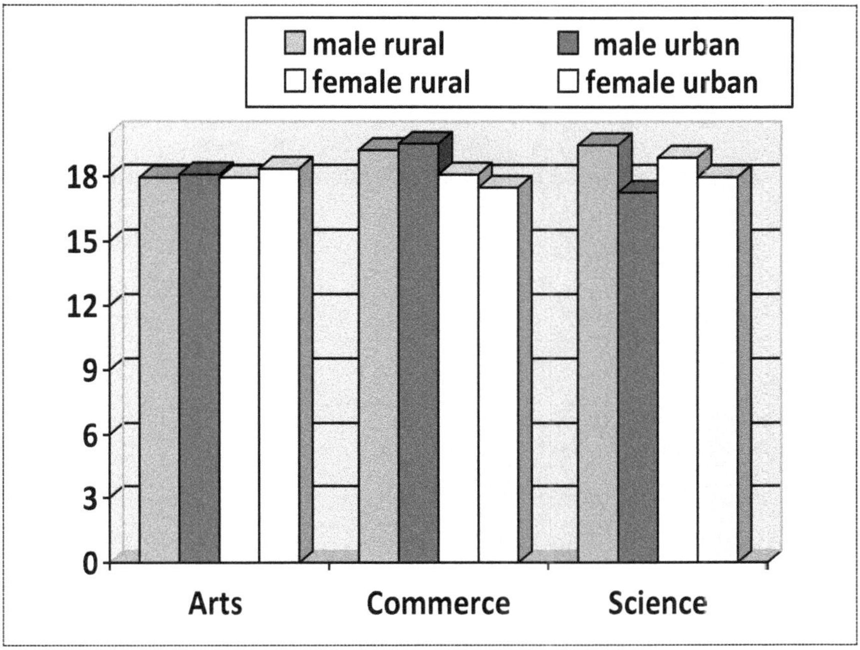

Figure No.49

The bars chart of interaction between the types of faculty, sex and area variables on Environmental mastery a part of mental health.

It is observed from the table No.**4.9.15** that the Interaction F for types of Faculty, Sex variables and Area variables on Environmental mastery a part of mental health. F value was **2.14**, which was not significance at **0.05** levels. Hence, the **Ho_{49}** was not rejected at 0.05 levels and it could be said that there was no significant mean difference between Sex variables and Area variables & their Environmental mastery a part of mental health score.

It could be seen from the table 4.9.16 and figure No.49 the **L.S.D.** for interaction between the Types of faculty, Sex variables and Area variables on Environmental mastery a part of mental health, that we seen the result and said that most of pairs are significance at 0.05 levels. We also said highest mean difference between $A_2B_1C_2$vs. $A_3B_2C_1$ (commerce male urban students vs. science female rural students) was **2.25**, so it can said that it was big difference.

Ho_{50}: There is no Correlation between Internet Addiction and Mental Health.

Table No 4.10
The correlation between Internet Addiction and Mental Health

Variables	N	Mean	r
Internet Addiction	720	28.04	**-0.41****
Mental Health.	720	37.53	

Critical Value for significance of Pearson product moment coefficient of correlation **'r'** value **df=718, 0.05= 0.06 / 0.01= 0.07**

It is observed that the table no.**4.10** the correlation between Internet Addiction and Mental Health that **'r' value** = **(-0.41),** so it can say that there was significant correlation between the respondents of Internet Addiction and Mental Health. Here, the normal negative **r** value = **(-0.41),** which was significant at 0.01 levels. It concluded that there was negative normal correlation between Internet Addiction and Mental Health**.** It means that as Internet Addiction increases and Mental Health decreases.

Ho_{51}: There is no significance difference between joint and nuclear family on Internet addiction

Table 4.11
t value of types of family on Internet addiction

Sr.No.	Type of Family	N	Mean	S.D.	't'	Significance
1	Joint	486	42.50	9.76	**2.71**	**0.01**
2	Nuclear	234	44.25	8.94		

Significance Levels 0.05=1.96 / 0.01=2.58

It observed from table no. 4.11 that the mean and S.D. of joint family was 42.50 and 9.76, the mean and S.D. of nuclear family was 44.25 and 8.94.So calculated t value is 2.71.It was significant at level of 0.01.This result also reveal that Nuclear family was higher Internet addict than Joint family.

Ho_{52}: There is no significance difference between joint and nuclear family on Mental Health

Table 4.12

t value of types of family on Mental Health

Sr.No.	Type of Family	N	Mean	S.D.	't'	Significance
1	Joint	486	94.19	10.68	**2.04**	**0.05**
2	Nuclear	234	96.53	11.25		

Significance Levels 0.05=1.96 / 0.01=2.58

It observed from table no. 4.11 that the mean and S.D. of joint family was 94.19 and 10.68, the mean and S.D. of nuclear family was 96.53 and 11.25,So calculated t value is 2.04.It was significant at level of 0.05.This result also reveal that Nuclear family was good Mental Health than Joint family.

Chapter 05: Research Report

5.1 Introduction

This section brings out the entire summary of the research, the conclusions made out of the investigation and recommendations for further Research.

5.2 Research Summary

The aim of present study is a study of Internet Addiction and Mental Health among the students of Arts, Commerce and Science faculty. So here according to sample has been selected **3x2x2 factorial design.**

The respondents of present study shall be 720 Subjects, randomly selected from different colleges of Gandhinagar, Ahmadabad of Gujarat state. The total sample consisting of **720** Subjects out which 24**0** are from Arts faculty**, 240** are from Commerce faculty and rest **240** are from Science faculty. In subjects of **720** out of which **360** are male and **360** are female. In subjects of **720** out of which **360** are rural students and 36**0** are urban students.

In this research two tests were administrated individually as well as on faculty of Arts , Commerce and Science students, In this research questionnaire including personal data sheet, Internet Addiction test was developed by **Kimbal Young** and adopted by **Mittal Vekariya ,** Mental Health Questionnaire was developed by **Dr.D.J.Bhatt and Gita R.Gida.** Before trying to do a questionnaire, study topics and ask them to carefully read topics and follow them. So the data collection was completed then **'F'** test **ANOVAs** was applied to check significance difference of main and internal effect of Arts, Commerce and Science faulty students also use the **L.S.D.** (least significance difference) was used to check significance difference of main and internal interaction of students of Arts, Commerce and Science faculty, and then **'r'** was used to check the correlation of Internet Addiction and Mental Health.

5.3 Research Conclusions

Based on the study, the following conclusions were as under:

1. There is significance difference of Internet Addiction based on types of Faculty variables.

2. There is significance difference of Internet Addiction based on Sex variables.
3. There is no significance difference of Internet Addiction based on Area variables.
4. There is no significance difference of Internet Addiction based on Interaction for types of Faculty and Sex variables.
5. There is no significance difference of Internet Addiction based on interaction for types of Faculty and Area variables.
6. There is no significance difference of Internet Addiction based on interaction for Sex and Area variables.
7. There is significance difference of Internet Addiction based on interaction for types of Faculty, Sex and Area variables.
8. There is significance difference of Mental Health based on types Faculty variables.
9. There is significance difference of Mental Health based on Sex variables.
10. There is significance difference of Mental Health based on Area variables.
11. There is no significance difference of Mental Health based on Interaction for types of Faculty and Sex variables.
12. There is significance difference of Mental Health based on Interaction for types of Faculty and Area variables.
13. There is no significance difference of Mental Health based on Interaction for Sex and Area variables.
14. There is no significance difference of Mental Health based on Interaction for types of Faculty, Sex and Area variables.
15. There is significance difference of Perception Reality a part of mental health based on types of Faculty variables.

16. There is significance difference of Perception Reality a part of mental health based on Sex variables.

17. There is no significance difference of Perception Reality a part of mental health based on Area variables.

18. There is no significance difference of Perception Reality a part of mental health based on interaction for types of Faculty and Sex variables.

19. There is significance difference of Perception Reality a part of mental health based on interaction for types of Faculty and Area variables.

20. There is no significance difference of Perception Reality a part of mental health based on interaction for Sex and Area variables.

21. There is no significance difference of Perception Reality a part of mental health based on interaction for types of Faculty, Sex and Area variables.

22. There is significance difference of Integration a part of mental health based on types of Faculty variables.

23. There is no significance difference of Integration a part of mental health based on type Sex variables.

24. There is significance difference of Integration a part of mental health based on types of Area variables.

25. There is no significance difference of Integration a part of mental health based on interaction for types of Faculty and Sex variables.

26. There is significance difference of Integration a part of mental health based on interaction for types of Faculty and Area variables.

27. There is no significance difference of Integration a part of mental health based on interaction for Interaction for Sex, Area variables.

28. There is no significance difference of Integration a part of mental health based on interaction for types of Faculty, Sex and Area variables.

29. There is no significance difference of Positive-self evolution a part of mental health based on types of faculty variables.

30. There is significance difference of Positive-self evolution a part of mental health based on Sex variables.

31. There is significance difference of Positive-self evolution a part of mental health based on Area variables.

32. There is no significance difference of Positive-self evolution a part of mental health based on interaction for types of faculty and Sex variables.

33. There is significance difference of Positive-self evolution a part of mental health based on interaction for types of faculty and Area variables.

34. There is no significance difference of Positive-self evolution a part of mental health based on interaction for Sex and Area variables.

35. There is no significance difference of Positive-self evolution a part of mental health based on interaction for types of faculty, Sex and Area variables.

36. There is no significance difference of Group Oriented Attitudes a part of mental health based on types of faculty variables.

37. There is significance difference of Group Oriented Attitudes a part of mental health based on Sex variables.

38. There is no significance difference of Group Oriented Attitudes a part of mental health based on Area variables.

39. There is no significance difference of Group Oriented Attitudes a part of mental health based on interaction for types of faculty and Sex variables.

40. There is no significance difference of Group Oriented Attitudes a part of mental health based on interaction for types of faculty and Area variables.

41. There is no significance difference of Group Oriented Attitudes a part of mental health based on interaction for types of Sex and Area variables.

42. There is no significance difference of Group Oriented Attitudes a part of mental health based on interaction for types of faculty, Sex and Area variables.

43. There is significance difference of Environmental Mastery a part of mental health based on types of faculty variables.

44. There is significance difference of Environmental Mastery a part of mental health based on Sex variables.

45. There is significance difference of Environmental Mastery a part of mental health based on Area variables.

46. There is significance difference of Environmental Mastery a part of mental health based on interaction for types of faculty and Sex variables.

47. There is significance difference of Environmental Mastery a part of mental health based on interaction for types of faculty and Area variables.

48. There is no significance difference of Environmental Mastery a part of mental health based on interaction for Sex and Area variables.

49. There is no significance difference of Environmental Mastery a part of mental health based on interaction for types of faculty, Sex and Area variables.

50. There is negative Correlation between Internet Addiction and Mental Health.

51. There is significance difference between Joint and Nuclear family on Internet Addiction

52. There is significance difference between Joint and Nuclear family on Mental Health

5.4 Limitations of the study

We all are know that our research are depend on Human behaviors, So many Human behaviors (traits) are affect to in our research (e.g. nature, Prejudice, like-dislike, attitude etc.). So we can say that some limitations of social science research are as under;

1. Here total sample consisting of only **720** Subjects. Some definite places have been used in this study like Gandhinagar, Ahmedabad and Visnagar districts in Gujarat so that finding of the study can not to be generalized on large population.
2. The present research to method of collecting Data using only the Inventory method, no any scientific method are using for data collecting like as interview method, survey method, analytical method etc.
3. In the study, only selected dependent variables was choose like as Internet Addiction and Mental Health But we included some others dependent variables (e.g. Frustration, Adjustment, etc.)
4. In the study the sample have been selected in between 17-23 years. None those who are Lower and Upper Age.
5. The present study is only for regular college students.
6. In this present study choose only Arts, Commerce and Science college students but not medical, engineering and other faculty students.
7. The present study is a psychological study; we very well know that Psychology is a science of Behaviors. So our psychological researches are depending on Human behaviors and Human behaviors (traits) are affected to in our research (e.g. nature, Prejudice, like-dislike, attitude etc.) so present some limitation for this study but may be moreover limitation in this study.

5.5 Suggestions for this Study

The following suggestions were presented for further studies are as follows:

1. Choosing Areas of present study are only for Gandhinagar, Ahmedabad and Visnagar districts in Gujarat, so in the future, study criteria for area moreover than this study.
2. In this present study only selected variables like as Internet Addiction and Mental Health so the future studies are indicated that others variables (e.g., Frustration, Adjustment, Life satisfaction etc.)
3. In the present study to method of collecting Data using only the Inventory method, no any scientific method are using for data collecting so in the future study we getting the good result we would like as some others techniques like as interview method, survey method, analytical method etc.
4. The present study chooses the some type of college going students but in the future study the will choose students who study with distance university, diploma students.
5. In the future study researcher collect inventory data but some other personal information for research samples, researcher contact and meet to samples relative and family members.
6. A study could be conducted regarding personality differences among other faculty students like medical, engineering, IIT or other students.
7. Cross cultural and comparative study with different type of factors like Religion, Cast, and Type of family, size of family and education level could be challenging area for further study.
8. Last but not least, same study may be revised after five year and verify the results of the study.
9. Age group in this study was 17-23 in future age group will increase in years.

CPSIA information can be obtained
at www.ICGtesting.com
Printed in the USA
LVHW040245020323
740706LV00017B/1533

9 781806 792399